Somatic Exercises for Beginners

Overcome Stress, Chronic Pain, and Anxiety with 60+ Proven Techniques – a 28-Day Journey to Mind-Body Connection in 10 Minutes a Day | Includes Guided Video Tutorials

Author Name: Gary Rodriguel

Unlock Exclusive Content Today!

Get access to our exclusive bonus material by downloading it now. Dive deeper into the topics covered in the book and enhance your learning experience.

QR Code

(Add a page before the table of contents with QR Code and Link to download a Bonus. I will give you the link and QR Code.)

TABLE OF CONTENTS

INTRODUCTION 7

UNLOCKING THE SECRETS OF SOMATICS 7

The Somatic Pathway: Your First Steps Towards Healing 7

Navigating This Book: Tools and Insights for Your Journey 8

The Healing Power of Awareness: An Overview of Somatic Benefits 10

CHAPTER 1 13

THE SOMATIC FOUNDATION 13

Bridging Mind and Body: The Core Principles of Somatics 13

Neurobiology and Healing:How Somatic Practices Rewire the Brain 15

CHAPTER 2 19

BREATHING LIFE INTO YOUR PRACTICE 19

Breath as Therapy: Techniques That Transform 19

BREATHING PATTERNS 21

Diaphragmatic Breathing 21

Box Breathing (Four-Square Breathing) 23

Segmented Breathing 24

Alternate Nostril Breathing (Nadi Shodhana) 25

Ocean Breath (Ujjayi Pranayama) 26

Breath of Fire (Kapalabhati) 28

4-7-8 Breathing 29

Lion's Breath (Simhasana) 30

Humming Bee Breath (Bhramari) 31

Equal Breathing (Sama Vritti) 33

Resonance Breathing 34

Sitali Breath 35

3-Part Breathing (Dirga Pranayama) 36

Circular Breathing 37

Visualization Breath 39

CHAPTER 3 41

EXERCISE FOR STRESS AND ANXIETY RELIEF 41

Progressive Muscle Relaxation 41

Movement Meditation 42

Grounding through Body Contact 44

Mindfulness and Presence Exercises 45

Guided Visualization for Relaxation 47

Somatic Sighing 49

Somatic Breath Counting 50

Humming 52

Somatic Writing 53

CHAPTER 4 .... *55*

EXERCISE FOR EMOTIONAL RESILIENCE AND REGULATION *55*

Body Scan Meditation 55

Eye Palming 56

Grounding Exercises 58

Mindful Walking 59

Somatic Visualization 61

Emotional Regulation Exercises 62

Leg Shaking 64

Butterfly Pose 65

CHAPTER 5 .... *67*

EXERCISE FOR PAIN RELIEF *67*

Slow Neck Rotations 67

Lateral Neck Tilts with Manual Resistance 68

Deep Breathing in Child's Pose 69

Myofascial Massage with Tennis Ball under the Neck 71

Controlled Breathing in Cat-Cow Pose 72

Circular Shoulder Movements to Relieve Tension 74

PILATES EXERCISES FOR LOWER BACK PAIN REDUCTION *76*

Psoas Release Exercise 76

Self-Massage 78

CHAPTER 6 .... *81*

EXERCISE FOR OVERCOMING TRAUMA *81*

Trauma Release Exercises 81

Pendulation Movements 83

Grounding and Centering Exercises 85

Body-Mind Connection Exercises 86

Tai Chi Movements 87

Spinal Twists 89

Pelvic Tilts 91

CHAPTER 7...**95**

EXERCISE FOR POSTURE AND FLEXIBILITY..**95**

Dynamic Stretching 95

Fluid and Circular Movements 98

Spinal Relaxation and Stretching Practices 100

Balance and Coordination Exercises 100

Spinal Twists 103

Rolling Down the Spine...105

Child's Pose...107

CHAPTER 8...**109**

THE 28-DAY SOMATIC CHALLENGE (BONUS CHAPTER) **109**

A 28 Day-by-Day Guide to Transforming Your Body and Mind with 10 minutes per day (Bonus) 109

Week-by-Week Progress Tracker (Somatic Exercise Workbook) (Bonus) 114

CONCLUSION **117**

CONTINUING YOUR SOMATIC JOURNEY **117**

Embodying the Lessons Learned..117

UNLOCKING THE SECRETS OF SOMATICS

The Somatic Pathway: Your First Steps Towards Healing

The somatic pathway is an invitation to reconnect with your body and uncover the deep wisdom it holds. This journey is not just about understanding trauma but about feeling it, processing it, and ultimately healing from it through your body's innate capacity for recovery. The somatic pathway begins with the recognition that trauma is stored in the body, manifesting as physical sensations, tension, and a myriad of symptoms that can disrupt your life. By tuning into these bodily experiences, you start to access the core of your trauma, allowing for a profound and transformative healing process.

Your first steps on this pathway involve developing a heightened awareness of your body's sensations. This means paying attention to the subtle cues your body provides—sensations of tightness, warmth, cold, tingling, or even numbness. These sensations are not random; they are your body's way of communicating unresolved stress and trauma. By learning to listen to these signals without judgment, you begin to honor your body's experience and create a safe space for healing.

As you move forward, it's crucial to cultivate a sense of safety within yourself. Trauma often disrupts our sense of safety, leaving us feeling vulnerable and disconnected. Creating a safe environment, both internally and externally, helps your body relax and start the healing process. This might involve finding a quiet, comfortable place where you can practice your somatic exercises or surrounding yourself with supportive and understanding people. Developing a compassionate relationship with yourself is key, as it fosters trust and encourages your body to release stored trauma.

Engaging in somatic exercises is another vital step. These exercises, such as gentle movement, deep breathing, and grounding techniques, are designed to help you release tension and reconnect with your body. They empower you to regulate your nervous system, reduce symptoms of trauma, and foster a sense of calm and stability. Through consistent practice, you will notice gradual changes in how your body responds to stress and trauma, feeling more grounded and resilient over time.

Understanding the science behind somatic experiencing can also enhance your journey. Somatic practices are rooted in neuroscience and the understanding of how trauma affects the brain and body. This knowledge provides a foundation for why these techniques are effective, giving you confidence in the process and motivating you to continue. Learning about the autonomic nervous system, the role of the vagus nerve, and the body's natural ability to heal can be empowering and reassuring as you navigate your healing journey.

Remember that healing is not a linear process. It's normal to encounter challenges and setbacks along the way. Be patient with yourself and acknowledge the progress you make, no matter how small it may seem. Each step you take on the somatic pathway brings you closer to a state of wholeness and well-being. With time, persistence, and compassion, you can unlock the secrets of somatics and discover the transformative power of healing from within.

Navigating This Book: Tools and Insights for Your Journey

Welcome to this transformative guide on somatic experiencing and trauma recovery. As you embark on this journey, it's essential to have a clear understanding of how to navigate this book to make the most of the tools and insights provided. This book is designed to be your companion, offering guidance, support, and practical techniques to help you heal from trauma and reconnect with your body.

In the following chapters, you will be introduced to the foundational concepts of somatic experiencing. We will delve into the science behind trauma and its impact on the body, helping you understand why traditional talk therapies might not have been sufficient for your healing. This knowledge lays the groundwork for the somatic techniques you will learn, providing you with a solid foundation to build upon.

Each chapter is structured to provide a blend of theoretical understanding and practical application. You will find detailed explanations of key concepts, followed by step-by-step instructions for exercises and techniques. These exercises are designed to be accessible and easy to integrate into your daily life, helping you develop a consistent practice that supports your healing journey.

Throughout the book, you will encounter real-life stories and case studies. These narratives are included to illustrate the transformative power of somatic experiencing and to offer hope and inspiration. Seeing how others have navigated their paths to healing can be incredibly empowering and can provide you with the motivation to continue on your own journey.

As you work through the exercises and techniques, it's important to approach them with an open mind and a compassionate heart. Healing from trauma is a deeply personal process, and it's normal to experience a range of emotions along the way. Be gentle with yourself and give yourself permission to move at your own pace. There is no right or wrong way to engage with these practices—what matters most is that you listen to your body and honor its signals.

This book also emphasizes the importance of creating a supportive environment for your healing. You will find suggestions for building a safe space, both physically and emotionally, where you can practice the techniques and reflect on your experiences. Additionally, we encourage you to seek out community support, whether through therapy, support groups, or connecting with others who are on a similar journey. Healing is often enhanced when we feel connected and supported by others.

Throughout your reading, you may come across terms or concepts that are new to you. A glossary is provided at the end of the book to help clarify these terms and ensure you have a thorough understanding of the material. If at any point you feel overwhelmed or uncertain, take a moment to pause and reflect. Return to the exercises and techniques that resonate most with you, and remember that this journey is about progress, not perfection.

Lastly, this book is meant to be a dynamic resource. You may find it helpful to revisit certain chapters or exercises as you progress on your healing journey. The insights and tools provided here are designed to support you at different stages of your recovery, offering ongoing guidance and inspiration.

We are honored to be part of your healing journey and are here to support you every step of the way. May this book serve as a beacon of hope and a practical guide, helping you unlock the secrets of somatics and discover the profound healing that lies within you.

The Healing Power of Awareness: An Overview of Somatic Benefits

Awareness is the cornerstone of somatic experiencing and a powerful tool in the journey toward healing from trauma. By cultivating a deeper awareness of your body and its sensations, you can begin to unravel the complex web of trauma stored within. This chapter explores the transformative benefits of developing awareness and how it can significantly impact your recovery process.

When you bring awareness to your body, you initiate a process of reconnection. Trauma often causes a disconnection between the mind and body, leaving you feeling detached and disoriented. By tuning into your bodily sensations, you start to bridge this gap, fostering a sense of unity and presence. This reconnection is the first step toward reclaiming your body as a safe and integral part of yourself.

One of the key benefits of heightened awareness is the ability to identify and release tension stored in the body. Trauma can cause chronic tension and holding patterns that contribute to physical pain and discomfort. Through mindful observation of your body's sensations, you can recognize areas of tightness and learn to gently release them. This process not only alleviates physical symptoms but also promotes a sense of relaxation and ease.

Awareness also plays a crucial role in regulating the nervous system. Trauma disrupts the natural balance of the nervous system, leading to states of hyperarousal or hypoarousal. By paying attention to your body's signals, you can learn to recognize when you are becoming overwhelmed or shutting down. With this knowledge, you can employ somatic techniques to bring your nervous system back into a state of equilibrium, enhancing your overall sense of stability and well-being.

Furthermore, developing body awareness enhances emotional regulation. Emotions are closely tied to physical sensations, and by becoming attuned to these sensations, you can better understand and manage your emotional responses. This heightened awareness allows you to process emotions more effectively, reducing the intensity and duration of emotional distress. Over time, this can lead to greater emotional resilience and a more balanced emotional state.

Another profound benefit of somatic awareness is its impact on self-awareness and self-compassion. As you become more attuned to your body, you gain a deeper understanding of your experiences and reactions. This increased self-awareness fosters a sense of compassion and empathy toward yourself. You begin to see your reactions not as flaws or weaknesses but as understandable responses to past trauma. This shift in perspective is empowering and can significantly enhance your self-esteem and self-worth.

Awareness also facilitates the release of trauma through the completion of self-protective responses. Trauma often interrupts the natural fight, flight, or freeze responses, leaving these energies trapped in the body. By bringing mindful awareness to these sensations, you can allow these incomplete responses to resolve, freeing the trapped energy and facilitating healing. This process can lead to a profound sense of relief and liberation as your body completes what it was unable to during the traumatic event.

In addition to these benefits, developing somatic awareness can improve your overall health and well-being. Chronic stress and trauma can take a toll on the body, contributing to various health issues. By regularly practicing somatic awareness, you can reduce stress levels, improve sleep, boost immune function, and enhance overall physical health. This holistic approach to healing acknowledges the interconnectedness of the mind and body, promoting overall wellness.

As you continue to develop your awareness, you will likely experience a greater sense of presence and mindfulness in your daily life. This increased presence allows you to fully engage with your experiences, fostering a deeper connection to yourself and others. It also enhances your ability to enjoy and appreciate the present moment, contributing to a richer and more fulfilling life.

The healing power of awareness lies in its ability to reconnect you with your body, regulate your nervous system, enhance emotional and self-awareness, and promote overall health and well-being. By cultivating somatic awareness, you unlock a powerful tool for healing and transformation, paving the way for a brighter and more resilient future.

CHAPTER 1

THE SOMATIC FOUNDATION

Bridging Mind and Body: The Core Principles of Somatics

Understanding the core principles of somatics is essential for grasping how this approach bridges the gap between mind and body, leading to profound healing and transformation. Somatics recognizes that the mind and body are not separate entities but are intricately interconnected. This holistic view is central to somatic experiencing, a therapeutic approach that emphasizes bodily awareness as a pathway to resolving trauma.

At the heart of somatics is the principle of embodiment, which involves fully inhabiting and experiencing your body. Trauma can cause a sense of disconnection from the body, making it difficult to feel present and grounded. Embodiment practices aim to restore this connection, allowing you to feel more attuned to your bodily sensations and responses. By engaging with your body in this way, you can access the deep wisdom it holds and begin to understand how past traumas have shaped your physical and emotional experiences.

Another fundamental principle is the recognition of the body's innate capacity for healing. Somatics is grounded in the belief that the body has a natural ability to heal from trauma, given the right conditions. This healing potential is often hindered by the chronic stress and tension that trauma imposes. Somatic practices focus on creating a supportive environment where the body can relax and activate its self-healing mechanisms. This involves fostering a sense of safety, both within oneself and in one's surroundings, which is crucial for the healing process.

Somatics also emphasizes the importance of sensory awareness. This principle involves paying close attention to the physical sensations in your body, which can provide valuable insights into your emotional and psychological state. Sensory awareness helps you recognize patterns of

~ 13

tension and discomfort that are linked to unresolved trauma. By becoming more aware of these sensations, you can begin to address and release the underlying trauma, leading to greater physical and emotional freedom.

A key aspect of somatic experiencing is the concept of titration, which refers to the gradual and controlled release of traumatic energy. Rather than confronting traumatic memories and sensations all at once, somatics encourages a slow and steady approach. This helps prevent overwhelm and allows the body to integrate and process the trauma at a manageable pace. Titration ensures that the healing process is gentle and sustainable, reducing the risk of retraumatization.

Another core principle is pendulation, which involves moving between states of distress and safety. In somatic experiencing, you learn to oscillate between focusing on traumatic sensations and then returning to a state of comfort and stability. This back-and-forth movement helps expand your capacity to tolerate and process trauma while maintaining a sense of safety. Pendulation allows you to build resilience and gradually increase your ability to cope with traumatic memories and sensations.

The principle of grounding is also central to somatics. Grounding techniques are designed to help you connect with the present moment and your physical body. These practices can include deep breathing, mindfulness, and physical exercises that anchor you in the here and now. Grounding is particularly important for individuals who experience dissociation, a common response to trauma that involves feeling disconnected from reality. By grounding yourself, you can counteract dissociation and develop a stronger sense of presence and stability.

Finally, the principle of integration is vital in somatic experiencing. Integration involves bringing together the fragmented aspects of your experience into a coherent whole. Trauma often causes a sense of fragmentation, where different parts of yourself feel disconnected or in conflict. Somatic practices aim to integrate these parts, fostering a sense of unity and wholeness. This process can lead to a deeper understanding of yourself and your experiences, promoting long-term healing and growth.

The core principles of somatics—embodiment, the body's innate healing capacity, sensory awareness, titration, pendulation, grounding, and integration—work together to bridge the mind and body. By engaging with these principles, you can unlock the transformative potential of somatic experiencing, leading to profound healing and a renewed sense of connection and well-being.

Neurobiology and Healing: How Somatic Practices Rewire the Brain

The neurobiological underpinnings of somatic practices provides profound insights into how these methods facilitate healing from trauma. Trauma can significantly alter the brain's structure and function, leading to persistent symptoms such as hyperarousal, anxiety, and emotional dysregulation. However, the brain's remarkable plasticity—its ability to change and adapt—offers hope for recovery. Somatic practices harness this plasticity, promoting neural rewiring and fostering resilience and healing.

Trauma often triggers changes in the brain's limbic system, particularly the amygdala, hippocampus, and prefrontal cortex. The amygdala, responsible for processing emotions and detecting threats, becomes hyperactive, leading to heightened fear and anxiety responses. The hippocampus, which is crucial for forming and retrieving memories, can shrink under chronic stress, impairing its function and contributing to fragmented and intrusive memories. The prefrontal cortex, responsible for higher-order thinking and emotional regulation, can become underactive, leading to difficulties in managing emotions and impulses.

Somatic practices help to counteract these effects by engaging the body and mind in ways that promote neural integration and regulation. One key mechanism through which somatic practices facilitate healing is the activation of the parasympathetic nervous system, often referred to as the "rest and digest" system. By engaging in activities that promote relaxation and bodily awareness, such as deep breathing, mindful movement, and gentle touch, you can stimulate the parasympathetic nervous system. This activation helps to calm the amygdala, reduce stress hormone levels, and create a sense of safety and relaxation.

Another important aspect of somatic practices is their ability to enhance interoception, the awareness of internal bodily sensations. Interoception is mediated by the insular cortex, a region of the brain that plays a crucial role in integrating sensory information and emotional experiences. By increasing interoceptive awareness through somatic exercises, you can improve the communication between the body and brain. This enhanced connection helps to regulate emotional responses and foster a greater sense of self-awareness and emotional resilience.

Somatic practices also promote the process of neuroplasticity by encouraging the formation of new neural pathways. When you engage in repetitive, mindful movements or somatic exercises, you strengthen the connections between neurons, making these pathways more robust. Over time, this can lead to the reorganization of brain networks involved in emotional regulation, stress response, and memory processing. For instance, regularly practicing grounding exercises can help to strengthen the neural circuits associated with feelings of safety and stability, reducing the impact of traumatic triggers.

Additionally, somatic practices often involve the completion of incomplete self-protective responses, which are physiological reactions that were interrupted or suppressed during the traumatic event. Completing these responses can help to discharge the residual energy associated with trauma, leading to a reduction in symptoms such as hyperarousal and intrusive memories. This process is mediated by the brain's subcortical structures, including the basal ganglia, which are involved in motor control and the execution of habitual behaviors. By allowing these self-protective responses to complete, you can facilitate the reorganization of neural circuits and promote a sense of resolution and healing.

The role of the vagus nerve, a critical component of the parasympathetic nervous system, is also significant in somatic healing. The vagus nerve influences heart rate, digestion, and various other bodily functions. Somatic practices, such as deep breathing and vocalization, can stimulate the vagus nerve, promoting a state of calm and relaxation. This vagal tone is associated with improved emotional regulation, social connection, and overall well-being.

Furthermore, engaging in somatic practices can lead to the release of neurochemicals that support brain health and emotional well-being. Activities that promote physical movement and relaxation can increase the production of endorphins, which are natural painkillers and mood enhancers. Additionally, practices that foster social connection and safety can boost levels of oxytocin, a hormone that enhances feelings of trust and bonding.

Somatic practices offer a powerful means of healing from trauma by harnessing the brain's plasticity and promoting neural rewiring. Through the activation of the parasympathetic nervous system, enhancement of interoception, promotion of neuroplasticity, completion of self-protective responses, stimulation of the vagus nerve, and release of beneficial neurochemicals, somatic practices can profoundly impact brain function and support the recovery process. By integrating these practices into your healing journey, you can foster resilience, emotional regulation, and a deeper sense of connection between mind and body.

Dear Reader,

Thank you for taking the time to read the first chapter of "Somatic Exercises for Beginners Overcome Stress, Chronic Pain, and Anxiety with 60+ Proven Techniques – a 28-Day Journey to Mind-Body Connection in 10 Minutes a Day | Includes Guided Video Tutorials" Your journey towards better health is important to us, and we hope that the insights provided here have been helpful and inspiring.

Your feedback is invaluable to us. It helps us understand what works well and what can be improved, ensuring that we can provide the best possible content to support you and others on similar paths. By sharing your thoughts, you not only help us improve but also assist other readers in finding the right resources for their needs.

How You Can Share Your Review on Amazon.com:

- Go to the page where you found my book.
- Navigate to the 'Customer Reviews' section.
- Click on 'Write a customer review' to share your valuable insights.

Instant QR Code Access: Simply scan the QR code below with your smartphone to be directed to the Amazon review section.

CHAPTER 2

BREATHING LIFE INTO YOUR PRACTICE

Breath as Therapy: Techniques That Transform

Breathing is an essential, automatic function that sustains life, but it is also a powerful tool for healing and transformation. Breathwork, the conscious practice of controlling and manipulating the breath, has been used for centuries across various cultures to promote physical, emotional, and spiritual well-being. In the context of somatic experiencing and trauma recovery, breathwork techniques can help regulate the nervous system, release stored trauma, and foster a deeper connection between mind and body.

One of the fundamental principles of breathwork is its ability to activate the parasympathetic nervous system, which counteracts the stress response initiated by the sympathetic nervous system. When you are stressed or traumatized, your breathing often becomes shallow and rapid, a physiological response designed to prepare the body for fight or flight. However, this type of breathing can perpetuate feelings of anxiety and tension. By practicing deep, slow, and rhythmic breathing, you can stimulate the parasympathetic nervous system, inducing a state of calm and relaxation. This shift not only reduces stress levels but also supports the body's natural healing processes.

Diaphragmatic breathing, also known as belly breathing, is one of the most effective techniques for engaging the parasympathetic nervous system. This technique involves breathing deeply into the diaphragm rather than the chest, allowing the abdomen to rise and fall with each breath. To practice diaphragmatic breathing, sit or lie down in a comfortable position, place one hand on your chest and the other on your abdomen. Inhale deeply through your nose, allowing your abdomen to expand while keeping your chest relatively still. Exhale slowly through your mouth, feeling your abdomen contract. Repeat this process for several minutes, focusing on the sensation of your breath and the movement of your abdomen. This practice can help reduce anxiety, lower blood pressure, and promote a sense of grounding and stability.

Box breathing, also known as square breathing, is another powerful breathwork technique that can enhance mental clarity and emotional stability. Box breathing involves inhaling, holding the breath, exhaling, and holding the breath again, each for an equal count, typically four seconds. To practice box breathing, find a comfortable position and close your eyes if you feel safe doing so. Inhale through your nose for a count of four, hold your breath for a count of four, exhale through your mouth for a count of four, and hold your breath again for a count of four. Repeat this cycle for several minutes. Box breathing can help to calm the mind, increase focus, and bring balance to the nervous system.

Alternate nostril breathing, or Nadi Shodhana, is a technique rooted in yogic tradition that balances the left and right hemispheres of the brain and harmonizes the flow of energy within the body. To practice alternate nostril breathing, sit comfortably with your spine straight. Use your right thumb to close your right nostril and inhale deeply through your left nostril. Close your left nostril with your right ring finger, release your right nostril, and exhale through the right nostril. Inhale through the right nostril, close it with your thumb, and exhale through the left nostril. Continue this pattern for several minutes. This technique can reduce stress, improve respiratory function, and enhance mental clarity.

Breathwork can also involve more dynamic techniques, such as holotropic breathwork, which aims to access deeper layers of consciousness and facilitate emotional release. Holotropic breathwork involves rapid and deep breathing, often accompanied by evocative music, in a controlled setting. This practice can bring up intense emotions and memories, allowing for their expression and integration. Due to its powerful nature, holotropic breathwork should be practiced under the guidance of a trained facilitator.

Integrating breathwork into your daily routine can offer numerous benefits for trauma recovery. Regular practice can help to build resilience, improve emotional regulation, and enhance overall well-being. It's important to approach breathwork with curiosity and patience, allowing yourself to explore different techniques and find what works best for you. Over time, these practices can become a cornerstone of your healing journey, providing a reliable means of connecting with your body, calming your mind, and transforming your emotional landscape.

In conclusion, breathwork is a transformative therapeutic tool that can significantly enhance the process of trauma recovery. Techniques such as diaphragmatic breathing, box breathing, alternate nostril breathing, and holotropic breathwork offer practical and accessible ways to regulate the nervous system, release stored trauma, and foster a deeper mind-body connection. By incorporating these practices into your healing journey, you can harness the healing power of your breath and create lasting positive change in your life.

BREATHING PATTERNS

Diaphragmatic Breathing

Diaphragmatic breathing, also known as belly breathing or abdominal breathing, is a fundamental breathing pattern that promotes relaxation, reduces stress, and enhances overall well-being. This technique involves engaging the diaphragm, a dome-shaped muscle located at the base of the lungs, to facilitate deep and efficient breathing.

To practice diaphragmatic breathing:

1. **Find a Comfortable Position**: Sit or lie down in a comfortable position. You can place one hand on your chest and the other on your abdomen to feel the movement of your breath.

2. **Inhale Deeply Through Your Nose**: Take a slow and deep breath in through your nose. As you inhale, allow your abdomen to expand outward while keeping your chest relatively still. Imagine filling your belly with air like a balloon.

3. **Exhale Slowly Through Your Mouth**: Exhale slowly through your mouth or nose, letting your abdomen naturally deflate as the air leaves your lungs.

Benefits of Diaphragmatic Breathing:

- **Reduces Stress and Anxiety**: Diaphragmatic breathing activates the parasympathetic nervous system, promoting relaxation and reducing the body's stress response.

- **Improves Oxygenation**: By filling the lungs more fully with each breath, diaphragmatic breathing improves oxygen exchange and enhances respiratory efficiency.

- **Enhances Mind-Body Connection**: Focusing on the movement of the abdomen during diaphragmatic breathing increases awareness of bodily sensations, fostering a deeper connection between mind and body.

Applications:

- **Daily Practice**: Incorporate diaphragmatic breathing into your daily routine, especially during moments of stress or before sleep to promote relaxation.

- **Mindfulness and Meditation**: Use this technique during mindfulness practices or meditation to deepen your focus and cultivate present-moment awareness.

- **Stress Management**: Practice diaphragmatic breathing in stressful situations to maintain composure and reduce the impact of stress on your body and mind.

Box Breathing (Four-Square Breathing)

Box breathing, also known as four-square breathing, is a structured breathing technique that promotes relaxation, reduces stress, and enhances focus and clarity.

To practice box breathing:

1. **Find a Comfortable Position**: Sit or lie down in a relaxed position with your spine straight. Close your eyes if it feels comfortable for you.

2. **Inhale Deeply Through Your Nose**: Inhale slowly and deeply through your nose, counting to four as you fill your lungs with air. Feel your abdomen expand as you breathe in.

3. **Hold Your Breath**: Once you have inhaled fully, hold your breath for a count of four. Keep your lungs filled with air and maintain a sense of calm and control.

4. **Exhale Slowly Through Your Mouth**: Exhale slowly and completely through your mouth, counting to four as you release the air from your lungs. Feel your abdomen deflate as you breathe out.

Benefits of Box Breathing:

- **Calms the Nervous System**: Box breathing activates the parasympathetic nervous system, promoting relaxation and reducing the body's stress response.

- **Enhances Mental Clarity**: This structured breathing pattern helps clear the mind, improve concentration, and enhance cognitive function.

- **Reduces Anxiety and Tension**: By regulating your breathing and promoting rhythmic patterns, box breathing can alleviate feelings of anxiety and tension.

Applications:

- **Stress Management**: Use box breathing during stressful situations or before challenging tasks to maintain composure and reduce anxiety.

- **Mindfulness and Meditation**: Incorporate box breathing into mindfulness practices or meditation sessions to deepen relaxation and enhance focus.

Box breathing is a versatile and effective technique that can be practiced anywhere and anytime you need to calm your mind and relax your body.

Segmented Breathing

Segmented breathing, also known as segmented or segmented exhalation breathing, is a breathing technique that focuses on extending the exhalation phase of each breath. This practice can help promote relaxation, improve oxygenation, and enhance mindfulness.

To practice segmented breathing:

1. **Find a Comfortable Position**: Sit or lie down in a comfortable position with your spine straight. You can close your eyes if it helps you focus.

2. **Begin with a Deep Inhalation**: Inhale slowly and deeply through your nose, filling your lungs completely. Focus on expanding your chest and feeling the breath fill your abdomen.

3. **Exhale in Segments**: Exhale slowly and steadily through your mouth or nose in a series of short breaths or segments, rather than in one continuous breath. Divide your exhalation into three or four equal parts.

Benefits of Segmented Breathing:

- **Promotes Relaxation**: Segmenting the exhalation can help release tension and promote a sense of calm and relaxation.

- **Enhances Mindfulness**: By focusing on the segmented exhalation, you cultivate mindfulness and present-moment awareness.

- **Improves Respiratory Efficiency**: This technique encourages more complete exhalation, which can improve the efficiency of gas exchange in the lungs and enhance oxygenation.

Applications:

- **Stress Relief**: Use segmented breathing during stressful situations or when feeling anxious to promote relaxation and reduce tension.

- **Sleep Aid**: Practice segmented breathing before bedtime to relax your body and mind, promoting better sleep quality.

Segmented breathing is a flexible and accessible technique that can be adapted to suit your individual needs and preferences.

Alternate Nostril Breathing (Nadi Shodhana)

Alternate nostril breathing, also known as Nadi Shodhana in Sanskrit, is a traditional yogic breathing technique that balances the flow of energy in the body and harmonizes the left and right hemispheres of the brain.

To practice alternate nostril breathing:

1. **Find a Comfortable Position**: Sit in a comfortable cross-legged position or on a chair with your spine straight. Relax your shoulders and place your left hand on your left knee, palm facing upward.

2. **Prepare for Breathing**: Use your right hand. Place your right thumb on your right nostril and your right ring finger or pinky finger

on your left nostril. Your index and middle fingers can rest gently on your forehead between your eyebrows.

3. **Begin the Practice**: Close your right nostril with your right thumb and inhale deeply and slowly through your left nostril. Count to yourself as you breathe in, aiming for a smooth and controlled inhalation.

Benefits of Alternate Nostril Breathing:

- **Enhances Respiratory Function**: Practicing alternate nostril breathing improves respiratory efficiency and encourages deeper, more controlled breathing.

- **Supports Emotional Balance**: Regular practice can help regulate emotions, cultivate inner peace, and improve emotional resilience.

Applications:

- **Stress Reduction**: Use alternate nostril breathing during stressful situations or when feeling anxious to calm the mind and relax the body.

- **Meditation Practice**: Incorporate Nadi Shodhana into your meditation sessions to enhance concentration, mindfulness, and spiritual awareness.

Alternate nostril breathing is a powerful and accessible technique that can be integrated into your daily routine to promote holistic well-being. peace.

Ocean Breath (Ujjayi Pranayama)

Ocean Breath, known as Ujjayi Pranayama in Sanskrit, is a soothing and rhythmic yogic breathing technique characterized by a gentle sound resembling ocean waves.

To practice Ocean Breath:

1. **Find a Comfortable Position**: Sit in a cross-legged position or lie down on your back with your spine straight. Close your eyes softly if it feels comfortable.

2. **Begin with Deep Breathing**: Inhale deeply and slowly through your nose, filling your lungs completely. Feel your abdomen and chest expand as you breathe in.

3. **Engage the Throat**: Constrict the back of your throat slightly, as if you are fogging up a mirror with your breath. This creates a gentle "ha" sound in the throat.

Benefits of Ocean Breath (Ujjayi Pranayama):

- **Enhances Concentration**: The audible sound of Ocean Breath helps to anchor the mind and enhance focus, making it beneficial for meditation and mindfulness practices.

- **Promotes Relaxation**: The slow, deep breaths combined with the gentle sound calms the nervous system, reduces stress, and induces a sense of relaxation.

Applications:

- **Yoga Practice**: Incorporate Ujjayi Pranayama into your yoga practice to deepen your breath awareness, enhance flexibility, and create a meditative flow.

- **Stress Management**: Use Ocean Breath during stressful situations or before challenging tasks to maintain composure, reduce anxiety, and promote clarity of mind.

Ocean Breath (Ujjayi Pranayama) is a gentle yet powerful breathing practice that can be integrated into daily life to enhance overall well-being..

Breath of Fire (Kapalabhati)

Breath of Fire, known as Kapalabhati in Sanskrit, is an energizing and cleansing yogic breathing technique.

To practice Breath of Fire:

1. **Find a Comfortable Position**: Sit in a cross-legged position or on a chair with your spine straight and shoulders relaxed. Close your eyes softly if it feels comfortable.

2. **Begin with Deep Breathing**: Take a deep inhalation through your nose, filling your lungs completely. Exhale forcefully and sharply through your nose to expel air from your lungs. This exhalation should be active and quick, like a strong sigh.

3. **Establish the Rhythm**: After the forceful exhale, allow the inhalation to happen naturally and passively. The focus is on the exhalation; the inhalation should naturally follow as your diaphragm relaxes.

Benefits of Breath of Fire (Kapalabhati):

- **Energizes the Body**: Breath of Fire increases oxygen supply to the brain and stimulates the nervous system, creating a revitalizing effect on the body.

- **Cleanses the Respiratory System**: The rapid exhalations help clear the lungs of stale air and impurities, promoting respiratory health.

Applications:

- **Yoga Practice**: Incorporate Breath of Fire into your yoga practice to warm up the body, increase energy flow (prana), and prepare for more dynamic movements or asanas.

- **Stress Relief**: Use Kapalabhati during stressful situations or when feeling mentally fatigued to refresh and rejuvenate the mind.

Breath of Fire (Kapalabhati) is a powerful breathing technique that should be practiced with awareness and control.

4-7-8 Breathing

The 4-7-8 breathing technique is a simple yet effective relaxation exercise that promotes calmness, reduces stress, and aids in falling asleep.

To practice the 4-7-8 breathing technique:

1. **Find a Comfortable Position**: Sit or lie down in a comfortable position with your spine straight. You can close your eyes gently if it helps you relax.

2. **Place Your Tongue**: Rest the tip of your tongue against the ridge of tissue just behind your upper front teeth throughout the exercise. You will keep this tongue position during both the inhalation and exhalation phases.

3. **Start with Exhaling Completely**: Exhale completely through your mouth, making a whooshing sound.

4. **Inhale Quietly through Your Nose for a Count of 4**: Close your mouth and inhale quietly through your nose for a count of 4 seconds. During this inhalation, focus on filling your lungs with air and expanding your abdomen.

5. **Hold Your Breath for a Count of 7 Seconds**: After inhaling, hold your breath for a count of 7 seconds. Maintain a relaxed state and refrain from tensing your body.

6. **Exhale Completely through Your Mouth for a Count of 8 Seconds**: Exhale slowly and completely through your mouth, making a whooshing sound, for a count of 8 seconds.

Benefits of 4-7-8 Breathing Technique:

- **Promotes Relaxation**: The extended exhalation triggers the body's relaxation response, calming the mind and reducing stress and anxiety.

- **Improves Sleep Quality**: Practicing 4-7-8 breathing before bedtime can help induce sleep and improve sleep quality by promoting relaxation.

Applications:

- **Stress Relief**: Use the 4-7-8 breathing technique during stressful situations to regain composure and promote relaxation.

- **Sleep Aid**: Practice this technique before bedtime to calm the mind and prepare the body for sleep.

The 4-7-8 breathing technique is a versatile tool that can be practiced anywhere and anytime to promote relaxation, reduce stress, and enhance overall mental and emotional well-being.

Lion's Breath (Simhasana)

Lion's Breath, known as Simhasana Pranayama in Sanskrit, is a powerful yogic breathing exercise that releases tension, reduces stress, and promotes a sense of liberation and empowerment.

To practice Lion's Breath:

1. **Find a Comfortable Position**: Sit in a cross-legged position or kneel on your heels with your knees apart. Place your hands on your knees or thighs.

2. **Sit Up Straight**: Straighten your spine and relax your shoulders. Close your eyes softly if it feels comfortable, or keep them open with a soft gaze.

3. **Inhale Deeply through Your Nose**: Take a deep inhalation through your nose, filling your lungs completely. Expand your chest and abdomen as you breathe in.

Benefits of Lion's Breath (Simhasana Pranayama):

- **Relieves Tension**: The forceful exhalation and stretching of the tongue and face muscles release tension and tightness in the face, jaw, and throat.

- **Reduces Stress**: Lion's Breath activates the parasympathetic nervous system, promoting relaxation and reducing stress and anxiety levels.

- **Improves Vocal Resonance**: Regular practice can improve vocal resonance and clarity by strengthening the muscles involved in speech and expression.

- **Increases Energy**: The energizing effect of Lion's Breath can help combat fatigue and increase mental alertness and vitality.

Applications:

- **Stress Relief**: Use Lion's Breath during times of stress or anxiety to release tension and restore a sense of calmness and clarity.

- **Preparation for Speech or Performance**: Practice this technique before speaking in public or performing to alleviate nervousness and improve vocal confidence.

Lion's Breath (Simhasana Pranayama) is a rejuvenating and empowering breathing technique that can be practiced by individuals of all ages and fitness levels.

Humming Bee Breath (Bhramari)

Humming Bee Breath, known as Bhramari Pranayama in Sanskrit, is a calming and soothing yogic breathing technique that resembles the gentle humming of a bee.

To practice Humming Bee Breath:

1. **Find a Comfortable Position**: Sit comfortably in a cross-legged position or on a chair with your spine straight and shoulders relaxed. Close your eyes softly if it feels comfortable.

2. **Relax Your Facial Muscles**: Take a moment to relax your facial muscles, jaw, and tongue. Ensure your lips are gently closed and teeth are slightly apart throughout the practice.

3. **Inhale Deeply and Silently through Your Nose**: Take a slow and deep inhalation through your nose, filling your lungs completely. Feel your abdomen and chest expand as you breathe in.

Benefits of Humming Bee Breath (Bhramari Pranayama):

- **Reduces Stress and Anxiety**: The steady humming sound calms the mind, reduces stress hormones, and promotes a sense of relaxation and inner peace.

- **Enhances Mood**: Bhramari Pranayama uplifts the mood and helps alleviate symptoms of anger, frustration, and agitation.

Applications:

- **Mindfulness Practice**: Incorporate Bhramari Pranayama into your mindfulness or meditation practice to deepen relaxation and cultivate inner awareness.

- **Stress Management**: Use Humming Bee Breath during stressful situations or when feeling overwhelmed to quickly restore calmness and emotional balance.

Humming Bee Breath (Bhramari Pranayama) is a gentle yet powerful breathing practice that can be practiced by individuals of all ages and fitness levels.

Equal Breathing (Sama Vritti)

Equal Breathing, known as Sama Vritti Pranayama in Sanskrit, is a simple and calming yogic breathing technique that involves equalizing the length of inhalation and exhalation.

To practice Equal Breathing:

1. **Find a Comfortable Position**: Sit in a cross-legged position or lie down on your back with your spine straight and shoulders relaxed. Close your eyes gently if it feels comfortable.

2. **Establish a Smooth Breath Pattern**: Begin by breathing in and out through your nose. Take a few natural breaths to settle into your rhythm.

3. **Inhale for a Count of 4**: Inhale slowly and steadily through your nose for a count of 4 seconds. Feel your abdomen and chest expand as you breathe in.

Benefits of Equal Breathing (Sama Vritti Pranayama):

- **Balances the Mind**: Equalizing the breath helps to harmonize the activity of the brain's hemispheres, promoting mental equilibrium and clarity.

- **Reduces Stress and Anxiety**: This technique activates the parasympathetic nervous system, inducing relaxation, and reducing the production of stress hormones.

Applications:

- **Stress Management**: Use Equal Breathing during stressful situations or when feeling anxious to restore a sense of calmness and emotional balance.

- **Pre-sleep Routine**: Practice this technique before bedtime to relax the body and mind, preparing for restful sleep.

Equal Breathing (Sama Vritti Pranayama) is a gentle yet effective breathing practice suitable for practitioners of all levels.

Resonance Breathing

Resonance breathing, also known as coherent breathing or paced breathing, is a technique that involves breathing at a specific rate to synchronize with your natural respiratory rhythm.

To practice resonance breathing:

1. **Find a Comfortable Position**: Sit or lie down in a comfortable position with your spine straight. Close your eyes gently if it helps you relax.

2. **Begin with Natural Breathing**: Start by observing your natural breathing pattern for a few moments without trying to change it. Notice the rhythm and depth of your breath.

3. **Establish the Breathing Rate**: In resonance breathing, the goal is typically to breathe at a rate of 5 to 7 breaths per minute. This translates to inhaling for a count of about 5 to 7 seconds and exhaling for a similar duration.

4. **Breathe Deeply and Slowly**: Inhale slowly and deeply through your nose for a count of 5 to 7 seconds. Feel your abdomen and chest expand as you fill your lungs with air.

Benefits of Resonance Breathing:

- **Balances the Nervous System**: Resonance breathing helps balance the autonomic nervous system, promoting relaxation and reducing the body's stress response.

- **Enhances Emotional Regulation**: This technique improves emotional stability and resilience by fostering coherence between the heart rate variability and breathing rhythm.

Applications:

- **Stress Management**: Use resonance breathing during stressful situations to restore emotional equilibrium and reduce the impact of stress.

- **Mindfulness and Meditation**: Incorporate this technique into mindfulness or meditation practices to deepen relaxation, focus the mind, and enhance present-moment awareness.

Resonance breathing is a gentle and effective technique that can be practiced by individuals of all ages and fitness levels.

Sitali Breath

Sitali Breath (also known as Cooling Breath) is a pranayama technique designed to cool the body, calm the mind, and reduce stress.

To practice Sitali breath:

1. **Find a Comfortable Position**: Sit comfortably with your spine straight, either cross-legged on the floor or in a chair with your feet flat on the ground. Relax your shoulders and place your hands on your knees or in your lap.

2. **Tongue Positioning**: Either roll your tongue into a tube shape (if you can) or if you cannot roll your tongue, purse your lips to create a small O shape with your mouth.

3. **Inhale Slowly and Deeply**: Inhale deeply and slowly through the rolled tongue or pursed lips. Feel the coolness of the breath as it passes over your tongue or lips.

Benefits of Sitali Breath:

- **Cooling Effect**: Sitali breath has a natural cooling effect on the body, making it beneficial during hot weather or when experiencing internal heat.

- **Calmness and Relaxation**: This technique helps to calm the mind, reduce stress, and promote relaxation by focusing on the soothing sensation of the breath.

Applications:

- **Heat Relief**: Use Sitali breath during hot weather or when feeling overheated to cool down the body and maintain comfort.

- **Stress Reduction**: Practice this technique to reduce stress, anxiety, and tension by promoting a sense of calmness and relaxation.

Sitali breath is a simple and effective breathing technique that can be practiced by individuals of all ages and fitness levels.

3-Part Breathing (Dirga Pranayama)

3-Part Breathing, known as Dirga Pranayama in Sanskrit, is a foundational yogic breathing technique that promotes relaxation, enhances breath awareness, and increases oxygen intake throughout the body.

To practice 3-Part Breathing:

1. **Find a Comfortable Position**: Sit or lie down in a comfortable position with your spine straight. Close your eyes gently if it helps you relax.

2. **Begin with Deep Breathing**: Take a few natural breaths to settle into a relaxed rhythm. Place one hand on your abdomen and the other on your chest to feel the movement of each area as you breathe.

3. **Inhale into the Abdomen**: Begin by inhaling deeply through your nose. Direct the breath into your abdomen, allowing it to expand fully. Feel your belly rise and push against your hand.

4. **Expand into the Diaphragm**: Continue inhaling as you expand the breath into your diaphragm. Feel the middle part of your chest and sides expand outward, while keeping your abdomen gently engaged.

Benefits of 3-Part Breathing (Dirga Pranayama):

- **Promotes Relaxation**: 3-Part Breathing calms the mind, reduces stress, and promotes a sense of relaxation and well-being.

- **Increases Oxygenation**: By fully expanding the lungs, this technique enhances oxygen intake and improves respiratory efficiency.

- **Enhances Breath Awareness**: Practicing Dirga Pranayama increases awareness of the breath and fosters a deeper connection to the body's natural rhythms.

Applications:

- **Yoga Practice**: Incorporate 3-Part Breathing into your yoga practice as a foundational breathing technique to prepare for asanas (postures) and enhance breath control.

- **Stress Relief**: Use Dirga Pranayama during stressful situations to calm the mind and restore equilibrium.

3-Part Breathing (Dirga Pranayama) is a gentle and effective technique that can be practiced by individuals of all ages and fitness levels.

Circular Breathing

Circular breathing is a technique primarily used by musicians, especially wind instrument players, to sustain a continuous sound without interruption.

How Circular Breathing Works:

1. **Build Up Air in Cheeks**: Begin by inhaling deeply through your nose to fill your lungs completely. Hold your breath momentarily and then puff out your cheeks with the stored air.

2. **Exhale Using Stored Air**: While exhaling through your mouth to maintain a constant stream of air, simultaneously refill your lungs

by inhaling through your nose. This allows you to continue playing or producing sound without interruption.

Benefits and Applications:

- **Musical Performance**: Circular breathing enables musicians to play wind instruments continuously, creating seamless melodies and extended notes without breaks.

- **Breath Control**: Practicing circular breathing improves breath control and lung capacity, which is beneficial for both musicians and individuals interested in enhancing respiratory function.

Techniques for Learning Circular Breathing:

- **Puff Cheeks Technique**: Start by practicing puffing out your cheeks and releasing air while inhaling through your nose. Focus on maintaining a steady flow of air without pauses.

- **Using a Straw**: Practice exhaling through a straw into water while simultaneously inhaling through your nose. This helps develop the coordination needed for circular breathing.

Considerations:

- **Patience and Practice**: Learning circular breathing requires patience and consistent practice to master the coordination of inhaling and exhaling simultaneously.

- **Physical Endurance**: It may initially feel challenging to maintain consistent airflow, so building up endurance through regular practice is essential.

Circular breathing is a specialized technique that offers unique benefits for musicians and can also be adapted for therapeutic and mindfulness practices.

Visualization Breath

Visualization breath, also known as guided imagery breathing, combines deep breathing with mental imagery to promote relaxation, reduce stress, and enhance focus.

How to Practice Visualization Breath:

1. **Find a Quiet Space**: Sit or lie down in a comfortable position where you won't be disturbed. Close your eyes gently to aid in visualization.

2. **Deep Breathing**: Begin by taking a few slow, deep breaths to relax your body and calm your mind. Inhale deeply through your nose, filling your lungs with air, and exhale slowly through your mouth, releasing tension with each breath.

3. **Choose a Visualization**: Select a calming and pleasant image or scene that resonates with you. It could be a peaceful beach, a serene forest, a favorite place from your memories, or any scene that evokes feelings of relaxation and tranquility.

4. **Incorporate Breathing Rhythm**: As you continue to breathe deeply, synchronize your breath with the visualization.

5. **Enhance the Experience**: Engage all your senses in the visualization. Feel the warmth of the sun, hear the gentle waves, smell the scent of flowers, or experience any sensory details that enhance the realism of your mental imagery.

Benefits of Visualization Breath:

- **Stress Reduction**: Visualization breath helps to reduce stress and anxiety by promoting relaxation and calming the mind.

- **Enhanced Focus**: This technique improves concentration and mental clarity by engaging in focused mental imagery.

- **Emotional Regulation**: Practicing visualization breath can help regulate emotions, promote positive feelings, and cultivate a sense of inner peace.

Applications:

- **Stress Management**: Use visualization breath during stressful situations to restore inner balance and perspective.

- **Performance Enhancement**: Visualize success and positive outcomes before important events or performances to boost confidence and mental preparation.

Visualization breath is a versatile and effective technique that can be adapted to suit various situations and personal preferences.

CHAPTER 3
EXERCISE FOR STRESS AND ANXIETY RELIEF
Progressive Muscle Relaxation

Progressive Muscle Relaxation (PMR) is a technique that involves systematically tensing and then relaxing different muscle groups to promote physical relaxation and reduce stress and anxiety.

How to Practice Progressive Muscle Relaxation:

1. **Find a Quiet Space**: Sit or lie down in a comfortable and quiet environment where you can relax without interruptions.

2. **Deep Breathing**: Begin with a few deep breaths to center yourself and prepare for relaxation. Inhale deeply through your nose, hold briefly, and exhale slowly through your mouth.

3. **Progressive Tensing and Relaxing**: Follow these steps for each muscle group:

   Start with the Feet: Focus on your feet. Slowly curl your toes tightly for a few seconds, then release and let them relax completely. Feel the tension leaving your muscles as you exhale.

   Move to the Calves and Thighs: Gradually tense the muscles in your calves by pressing your heels down, hold briefly, then release and feel the relaxation spread up through your thighs.

   Engage the Hips and Abdomen: Tighten your abdominal muscles by pulling them in towards your spine. Hold briefly, then release completely as you exhale, allowing your stomach to rise naturally.

4. **Progress Through Muscle Groups**: Continue this process, systematically tensing and relaxing each major muscle group in your body, from your feet to your head. Focus on the sensations of tension and relaxation in each muscle group.

Benefits of Progressive Muscle Relaxation:

~ 41

- **Reduces Muscle Tension**: PMR helps to alleviate physical tension and tightness in the muscles, which often accompanies stress and anxiety.

- **Promotes Relaxation Response**: By systematically relaxing muscles, PMR triggers the body's relaxation response, leading to reduced heart rate, blood pressure, and overall stress levels.

- **Enhances Mind-Body Awareness**: Practicing PMR increases awareness of the mind-body connection, fostering mindfulness and relaxation.

Applications:

- **Stress Management**: Use PMR as a daily practice to manage and reduce stress levels, promoting overall well-being.

- **Anxiety Relief**: Incorporate PMR into your routine during times of heightened anxiety to induce relaxation and calmness.

- **Complementary Therapy**: PMR can be used alongside other relaxation techniques, such as deep breathing and meditation, to enhance relaxation and stress relief.

Progressive Muscle Relaxation is a simple yet powerful technique that can be practiced by anyone to promote physical relaxation, reduce muscle tension, and alleviate stress and anxiety.

Movement Meditation

Movement meditation is a practice that combines mindfulness and physical movement to cultivate awareness, relaxation, and a sense of inner peace.

How to Practice Movement Meditation:

1. **Choose Your Movement**: Select a simple and repetitive movement or activity that you enjoy and can perform mindfully. This could

include walking, tai chi, qigong, yoga flows, dancing, or any other form of gentle exercise.

2. **Find a Quiet Space**: Practice in a quiet environment where you can move freely without distractions. This could be indoors or outdoors, depending on your preference.

3. **Center Yourself**: Begin by standing or sitting comfortably. Close your eyes if it helps you to focus inward and connect with your breath.

4. **Connect with Your Breath**: Take a few deep breaths to center yourself. Inhale deeply through your nose, feeling your abdomen rise, and exhale fully through your mouth, releasing any tension or distractions.

Benefits of Movement Meditation:

- **Improves Body Awareness**: Regular practice increases awareness of body sensations, posture, and movement patterns, fostering greater mind-body connection.

- **Promotes Emotional Well-being**: Movement meditation can improve mood, boost energy levels, and promote a sense of inner peace and emotional balance.

Applications:

- **Daily Practice**: Incorporate movement meditation into your daily routine as a way to start or end your day mindfully.

- **Stress Relief**: Use movement meditation during times of stress or overwhelm to relax the body and calm the mind.

- **Spiritual Exploration**: Explore movement meditation as a spiritual practice to deepen your connection with yourself and the world around you.

Movement meditation offers a dynamic and accessible approach to mindfulness and relaxation, making it suitable for individuals of all fitness levels and ages. By integrating mindful movement into your life, you can cultivate a greater sense of peace, awareness, and well-being.

Grounding through Body Contact

Grounding through body contact is a technique that involves connecting with the present moment and enhancing a sense of stability and security by focusing on physical contact with surfaces or objects.

How to Practice Grounding through Body Contact:

1. **Sit or Lie Down**: Position yourself in a relaxed posture. You can sit on a chair, cushion, or lie down on a comfortable surface such as a bed or yoga mat.

2. **Feel the Surface**: Close your eyes if it helps you focus inward. Begin by noticing the physical contact between your body and the surface beneath you. Feel the weight of your body being supported by the chair, cushion, or ground.

3. **Notice Sensations**: Pay attention to the sensations where your body makes contact with the surface. Feel the texture, temperature, and firmness of the surface against your skin.

4. **Breathe Mindfully**: Take slow, deep breaths to center yourself and relax. Inhale deeply through your nose, allowing your abdomen to expand, and exhale fully through your mouth, releasing any tension or stress.

5. **Visualize Grounding**: Visualize roots extending from your body down into the ground, anchoring you securely like the roots of a tree. Imagine yourself drawing stability and strength from the earth.

Benefits of Grounding through Body Contact:

- **Reduces Anxiety and Stress**: Grounding techniques help to reduce feelings of anxiety and stress by promoting a sense of stability and security.

- **Increases Mindfulness**: By focusing on physical sensations and the present moment, grounding enhances mindfulness and awareness.

- **Enhances Emotional Regulation**: Practicing grounding through body contact can help regulate emotions and promote a sense of calmness and relaxation.

Applications:

- **Daily Practice**: Incorporate grounding through body contact into your daily routine to start or end your day with a sense of stability.

- **Anxiety Management**: Use this technique during moments of heightened anxiety or stress to calm your mind and body.

Grounding through body contact is a simple yet effective technique that can be practiced anywhere and anytime to promote relaxation, reduce anxiety, and foster a greater sense of well-being.

Mindfulness and Presence Exercises

Mindfulness and presence exercises are practices that cultivate awareness of the present moment, enhance mental clarity, and promote overall well-being. These exercises involve focusing attention on sensory experiences, thoughts, emotions, or bodily sensations without judgment.

How to Practice Mindfulness and Presence:

1. **Mindful Breathing**:

   Find a quiet place to sit comfortably.

   Close your eyes gently and bring your attention to your breath.

   Notice the sensation of the breath as it enters and leaves your body.

2. **Body Scan Meditation**:

Lie down on your back or sit comfortably in a relaxed position.

Close your eyes and bring awareness to different parts of your body, starting from your toes and moving upward.

3. **Mindful Walking**:

Find a quiet outdoor space or a spacious indoor area where you can walk comfortably.

Begin walking slowly and deliberately, focusing on each step you take.

4. **Observing Thoughts and Emotions**:

Sit quietly and observe your thoughts and emotions as they arise.

Notice the content of your thoughts and the feelings associated with them.

Benefits of Mindfulness and Presence Exercises:

- **Stress Reduction**: Mindfulness practices help reduce stress by focusing attention on the present moment rather than worries about the future or regrets about the past.

- **Improved Focus and Concentration**: Regular practice enhances cognitive function, allowing for better focus and concentration in daily activities.

- **Enhanced Well-being**: By fostering a deeper connection with the present moment, mindfulness and presence exercises promote overall mental and emotional well-being.

Applications:

- **Daily Routine**: Integrate mindfulness and presence exercises into your daily routine to start or end your day with a sense of clarity and calm.

- **Stress Management**: Use these practices during stressful moments or busy periods to regain focus and reduce anxiety.

- **Relationship Building**: Practice mindfulness to improve communication and presence in relationships, fostering deeper connections with others.

Mindfulness and presence exercises offer powerful tools for cultivating a greater sense of awareness, relaxation, and well-being in daily life.

Guided Visualization for Relaxation

Guided visualization for relaxation is a technique that uses mental imagery to promote relaxation, reduce stress, and enhance overall well-being. This practice involves creating vivid, sensory-rich images in the mind to evoke feelings of calmness, safety, and inner peace.

How to Practice Guided Visualization for Relaxation:

1. **Prepare for the Session**:

   Find a quiet and comfortable space where you can sit or lie down without distractions.

   Dim the lights or create a soothing atmosphere with soft music, candles, or essential oils if desired.

   Make sure you are in a relaxed position, such as sitting in a comfortable chair or lying down on a yoga mat or bed.

2. **Deep Relaxation**:

   Close your eyes and begin by taking a few deep breaths. Inhale deeply through your nose, allowing your abdomen to expand, and exhale fully through your mouth, releasing any tension or stress with each breath.

3. **Begin the Visualization**:

Imagine yourself in a peaceful and serene environment that brings you comfort and relaxation. This could be a beach, forest, garden, or any place where you feel safe and at ease.

4. **Explore Sensory Experiences**:

As you continue to visualize, explore different sensory experiences. For example, feel the warmth of the sun on your skin, listen to the **Embrace Feelings of Relaxation**:

Notice how your body responds to the guided visualization. Feel a sense of calmness, tranquility, and inner peace spreading throughout your body and mind.

Benefits of Guided Visualization for Relaxation:

- **Stress Reduction**: Guided visualization promotes relaxation by calming the mind and body, reducing stress hormones, and lowering blood pressure.

- **Enhanced Well-being**: Regular practice improves overall well-being by fostering a positive outlook, reducing anxiety, and promoting emotional resilience.

- **Improved Sleep**: Guided visualization before bedtime can help improve sleep quality by relaxing the body and mind, making it easier to fall asleep and stay asleep.

Applications:

- **Daily Practice**: Include guided visualization in your daily routine to start or end your day with relaxation and mental clarity.

- **Self-Care**: Practice guided visualization as a form of self-care to nurture your mental and emotional well-being.

Guided visualization for relaxation is a powerful tool for reducing stress, enhancing relaxation, and promoting overall well-being.

Somatic Sighing

Somatic sighing is a therapeutic technique that combines intentional deep breathing with the natural sigh reflex to promote relaxation, release tension, and enhance emotional well-being.

How to Practice Somatic Sighing:

1. **Find a Comfortable Position:**

   Sit or lie down in a comfortable position where you can fully relax and focus on your breathing.

2. **Deep Breathing Preparation:**

   Begin with a few deep breaths to settle into your body and connect with your breath. Inhale deeply through your nose, allowing your abdomen to expand fully.

   Exhale slowly and completely through your mouth, releasing any tension or tightness with each breath out.

3. **Introducing Somatic Sighing:**

   Once you are settled into your breath, introduce somatic sighing by taking a slightly deeper inhale than usual through your nose.

4. **Repeat and Allow Release:**

   Continue to practice somatic sighing at your own pace, allowing each sigh to be a deliberate release of tension and stress.

Benefits of Somatic Sighing:

- **Stress Reduction**: Somatic sighing helps to release physical and emotional tension, promoting relaxation and reducing stress levels.

- **Emotional Release**: By allowing for a deep exhale, somatic sighing can facilitate the release of pent-up emotions and promote emotional well-being.

- **Muscle Relaxation**: The act of sighing encourages the relaxation of muscles, particularly in the shoulders, chest, and diaphragm.

Applications:

- **Daily Practice**: Incorporate somatic sighing into your daily routine as a quick relaxation technique or as part of a longer mindfulness practice.

- **Stressful Situations**: Use somatic sighing during moments of stress or anxiety to quickly calm your mind and body.

- **Before Bedtime**: Practice somatic sighing before bedtime to unwind and promote a restful night's sleep.

Somatic sighing is a simple yet effective technique for promoting relaxation, releasing tension, and enhancing overall well-being.

Somatic Breath Counting

Somatic breath counting is a mindfulness practice that combines conscious breathing with counting to enhance awareness, focus the mind, and promote relaxation.

How to Practice Somatic Breath Counting:

1. **Find a Quiet Space**:

   Sit or lie down in a comfortable position where you can relax without distractions. Close your eyes gently if it helps you focus.

2. **Begin with Deep Breathing**:

   Take a few deep breaths to settle into your body and connect with your breath. Inhale deeply through your nose, allowing your abdomen to expand fully.

3. **Start Counting Your Breaths**:

Once you feel relaxed and centered, begin counting your breaths silently in your mind. Start with the number one.

4. **Continue the Counting Process**:

Inhale again deeply for a count of three, and exhale for a count of four.

5. **Conclude Mindfully**:

After completing your chosen number of breaths, gradually transition back to regular breathing.

Benefits of Somatic Breath Counting:

- **Enhanced Focus and Concentration**: Somatic breath counting helps sharpen your focus and concentration by directing attention to the present moment.

- **Stress Reduction**: By focusing on the breath, this practice promotes relaxation and reduces stress levels.

- **Mindfulness and Awareness**: Somatic breath counting cultivates mindfulness by anchoring awareness in the breath and fostering a non-judgmental presence.

Applications:

- **Stress Management**: Use somatic breath counting during stressful moments or when feeling overwhelmed to regain composure and clarity.

- **Before Sleep**: Practice somatic breath counting before bedtime to relax your mind and body, promoting a restful night's sleep.

Somatic breath counting is a versatile technique that can be customized to suit your preferences and needs.

Humming

Humming is a simple yet effective somatic technique that involves producing a continuous sound by gently exhaling through closed lips, creating a humming vibration in the head and chest.

How to Practice Humming:

1. **Find a Quiet Environment**:

   Choose a quiet space where you can sit comfortably without distractions. You may close your eyes if it helps you focus inward.

2. **Relax and Center Yourself**:

   Take a few deep breaths to settle into your body and relax any tension you may be holding. Inhale deeply through your nose and exhale fully through your mouth.

3. **Begin to Hum**:

   Close your lips gently and take a slow, deep breath in through your nose.

   As you exhale, create a humming sound by gently vibrating your vocal cords with closed lips. The sound should be steady and continuous.

4. **Feel the Vibrations**:

   Notice the vibrations created by the humming sound, particularly in your head and chest. Allow these vibrations to resonate throughout your body.

Benefits of Humming:

- **Relaxation**: Humming promotes relaxation by activating the parasympathetic nervous system, reducing stress levels, and calming the mind.

- **Resonance**: The vibrations produced during humming resonate in the head and chest, providing a soothing effect on the body and mind.

- **Mind-Body Connection**: Humming enhances the mind-body connection by focusing attention on the physical sensation of sound and vibration.

Applications:

- **Stress Relief**: Use humming during stressful situations to quickly calm your mind and relax your body.

- **Before Meditation or Sleep**: Practice humming before meditation or bedtime to quiet the mind and prepare for deep relaxation or sleep.

Humming is a gentle and accessible somatic practice that can be integrated into various contexts to promote relaxation, reduce stress, and enhance overall well-being.

Somatic Writing

Somatic writing is a therapeutic practice that integrates somatic experiencing principles with expressive writing techniques.

How to Practice Somatic Writing:

1. **Set an Intention**:

   Begin by setting an intention for your somatic writing practice. This could be to explore a specific emotion, gain insight into a particular situation, or simply to release pent-up feelings.

2. **Mindful Awareness**:

   Close your eyes and take a few deep breaths to center yourself. Bring your awareness to your body and notice any sensations or tensions you may be experiencing.

3. **Start Writing**:

Open your eyes and begin writing freely without worrying about grammar or structure. Let your thoughts flow onto the paper, allowing your emotions to guide the writing process.

4. **Explore Emotions**:

As you write, explore the emotions that arise. Describe how you feel without judgment or criticism. Allow yourself to express both positive and challenging emotions.

Benefits of Somatic Writing:

- **Emotional Release**: Somatic writing provides a safe outlet for expressing and releasing emotions stored in the body.

- **Self-Exploration**: By focusing on bodily sensations and emotions, somatic writing encourages deeper self-exploration and understanding.

- **Stress Reduction**: Engaging in somatic writing can reduce stress levels by helping to process and cope with challenging emotions.

Applications:

- **Daily Practice**: Incorporate somatic writing into your daily routine as a form of self-reflection and emotional processing.

- **Therapeutic Tool**: Use somatic writing in conjunction with therapy or counseling to enhance emotional awareness and healing.

- **Creative Expression**: Explore creative writing exercises that integrate somatic awareness to deepen your creative process.

Somatic writing is a powerful tool for anyone seeking to explore emotions, enhance self-awareness, and promote emotional healing self-discovery.

CHAPTER 4
EXERCISE FOR EMOTIONAL RESILIENCE AND REGULATION

Body Scan Meditation

Body scan meditation is a mindfulness practice that involves systematically scanning through different parts of the body, cultivating awareness of physical sensations, and promoting relaxation.

How to Practice Body Scan Meditation:

1. **Find a Comfortable Position**:

   Sit or lie down in a comfortable position where you can relax without distractions. Close your eyes gently if it helps you focus inward.

2. **Begin with Deep Breathing**:

   Take a few deep breaths to settle into your body and relax any tension. Inhale deeply through your nose and exhale fully through your mouth, releasing any tightness or stress.

3. **Start at the Feet**:

   Bring your attention to your feet. Notice any sensations such as warmth, pressure, or tingling. Allow your feet to relax with each breath.

4. **Progress Upwards**:

   Slowly move your attention upwards, to your ankles, calves, knees, and thighs. With each part of the body, take a moment to observe any sensations without judgment.

   If you notice any tension or discomfort, gently breathe into that area and allow it to soften.

Benefits of Body Scan Meditation:

- **Stress Reduction**: Body scan meditation promotes relaxation and reduces stress by systematically releasing tension from different parts of the body.

- **Mindfulness**: This practice enhances mindfulness by directing attention to the present moment and physical sensations.

- **Improved Sleep**: Practicing body scan meditation before bedtime can improve sleep quality by relaxing the body and quieting the mind.

Applications:

- **Stress Management**: Use body scan meditation during stressful moments to bring yourself back to a state of calm and clarity.

- **Mind-Body Connection**: Deepen your understanding of the mind-body connection by regularly practicing body scan meditation and noticing how your body responds to different emotions and situations.

Body scan meditation is a valuable tool for enhancing overall well-being, promoting relaxation, and cultivating mindfulness.

Eye Palming

Eye palming is a simple yet effective technique that helps relieve eye strain, reduce tension around the eyes, and promote overall relaxation

How to Practice Eye Palming:

1. **Find a Comfortable Position**:

   Sit comfortably in a chair or lie down on your back in a quiet, dimly lit room. Ensure you are in a relaxed position with your shoulders relaxed and your spine comfortably aligned.

2. **Warm Your Hands**:

Rub your palms together vigorously for about 10-15 seconds until they feel warm. This warmth will help soothe your eyes and enhance relaxation.

3. **Palming Technique**:

Close your eyes gently and place your warm palms over your eyes, cupping them gently without applying pressure. Your fingers should overlap on your forehead, and the heels of your hands should rest lightly on your cheekbones.

4. **Create Darkness**:

Position your hands so that they create a gentle pressure-free seal around your eyes, ensuring there's no pressure on your eyeballs. You should be able to blink freely.

Benefits of Eye Palming:

- **Relief from Eye Strain**: Eye palming helps relax the muscles around the eyes, reducing strain caused by prolonged visual tasks.
- **Promotes Relaxation**: The warmth and darkness created by palming promote relaxation of the entire body, not just the eyes.
- **Reduces Stress**: Taking a few minutes for eye palming can reduce overall stress levels by providing a moment of calm and relaxation.

Applications:

- **Screen Breaks**: Use eye palming during screen breaks at work or when studying to refresh your eyes and mind.
- **Before Bed**: Practice eye palming before bedtime to relax your eyes and prepare for restful sleep.
- **During Travel**: Use eye palming during long flights or car rides to alleviate eye strain and promote relaxation.

Eye palming is a convenient and effective technique that can be practiced anywhere to relieve eye strain and promote overall relaxation.

Grounding Exercises

Grounding exercises are techniques that help individuals connect with the present moment, increase awareness of their surroundings, and regain a sense of stability and calm.

How to Practice Grounding Exercises:

1. **5-4-3-2-1 Technique**:

   Name 5 things you can see: Look around and identify five objects or items in your immediate surroundings.

   Name 4 things you can touch: Pay attention to the sensation of touch. Identify four things you can physically touch or feel.

   Name 3 things you can hear: Listen closely to your surroundings. Identify three sounds you can hear, whether near or far.

   Name 2 things you can smell: Take a deep breath and notice any scents or smells around you. Name two distinct smells you can detect.

   Name 1 thing you can taste: Focus on your sense of taste. Identify one taste or flavor you are currently experiencing or recall a recent taste.

2. **Grounding through Breath**:

   Find a comfortable sitting or standing position. Close your eyes if it helps you focus inward.

3. **Body Scan**:

   Close your eyes and bring your attention to your body. Start with your feet and slowly move upward, noticing any sensations or tensions.

4. **Walking Barefoot (Earthing)**:

   Find a safe outdoor space where you can walk barefoot on natural surfaces such as grass, sand, or soil.

Benefits of Grounding Exercises:

- **Calming Effect**: Grounding exercises promote relaxation and reduce feelings of anxiety or overwhelm.

- **Enhanced Awareness**: These practices increase mindfulness and awareness of the present moment and surroundings.

Applications:

- **Stress Management**: Use grounding techniques during stressful moments to regain composure and restore a sense of balance.

- **Anxiety Relief**: Practice grounding exercises regularly to alleviate symptoms of anxiety and promote a sense of calm.

Grounding exercises are valuable tools for anyone seeking to enhance their sense of presence, reduce stress, and cultivate emotional well-being.

Mindful Walking

Mindful walking is a practice that combines the physical act of walking with mindfulness techniques, allowing you to be fully present and aware of each step and movement. This practice can help reduce stress, increase focus, and promote a sense of calm and grounding.

How to Practice Mindful Walking:

1. **Find a Quiet Space**:

   Choose a quiet and peaceful location where you can walk without distractions. It could be outdoors in nature, a park, or a quiet indoor space.

2. **Begin with Awareness**:

Stand still for a moment and bring your attention to your body. Feel the contact of your feet with the ground and notice your posture.

3. **Set Your Intention**:

Set an intention for your mindful walk, such as focusing on the sensations of walking, observing nature, or simply being present in the moment.

4. **Start Walking Slowly**:

Begin to walk at a slow and steady pace. Pay attention to each movement of your feet – the lifting, moving forward, and placing them back on the ground.

Benefits of Mindful Walking:

- **Enhanced Awareness**: This practice increases mindfulness and sensory awareness, allowing you to appreciate the details of your environment.

- **Improved Mood**: Regular practice of mindful walking can uplift your mood and improve overall emotional well-being.

- **Physical Exercise**: It provides gentle physical exercise, promotes circulation, and improves flexibility while engaging in mindfulness.

Applications:

- **Daily Routine**: Incorporate mindful walking into your daily routine as a form of active meditation and stress relief.

- **Break from Technology**: Use mindful walking as a break from screens and technology, allowing yourself to reconnect with nature and your senses.

- **Group Practice**: Invite friends or family to join you for a mindful walk, fostering connections and shared mindfulness experiences.

Mindful walking is a powerful practice that integrates movement with mindfulness, offering numerous benefits for physical and mental well-being.

Somatic Visualization

Somatic visualization is a therapeutic technique that utilizes the power of imagination to promote relaxation, reduce stress, and facilitate healing within the body and mind.

How to Practice Somatic Visualization:

1. **Find a Quiet Space**:

   Choose a quiet and comfortable space where you can sit or lie down without distractions. Close your eyes to enhance focus.

2. **Deep Relaxation**:

   Begin by taking several slow, deep breaths to relax your body and calm your mind. Allow any tension or stress to melt away with each exhale.

3. **Body Awareness**:

   Bring your awareness to different parts of your body. Notice any sensations, tensions, or areas of discomfort without judgment.

4. **Choose a Healing Image**:

   Select a soothing and healing image that resonates with you. It could be a peaceful landscape, a place of safety and comfort, or a symbol of healing and resilience.

5. **Visualize with Detail**:

   Begin to visualize this image in your mind's eye with as much detail as possible. Imagine the colors, shapes, textures, and sounds associated with this place or symbol.

6. **Engage Your Senses**:

Engage all your senses in the visualization process. Notice how the image feels, smells, sounds, and even tastes in your imagination.

Benefits of Somatic Visualization:

- **Pain Management**: Visualization techniques have been shown to help manage chronic pain and discomfort by altering perceptions and responses to physical sensations.

- **Enhanced Well-Being**: Regular practice of somatic visualization can contribute to overall well-being by promoting a positive mindset and enhancing self-awareness.

Applications:

- **Preparation for Challenges**: Visualize positive outcomes before stressful events or challenges to enhance confidence and mental preparation.

Somatic visualization is a versatile and powerful technique that taps into the mind-body connection to support healing and well-being.

Emotional Regulation Exercises

Emotional regulation exercises are practices designed to help individuals manage and modulate their emotional responses effectively.

How to Practice Emotional Regulation Exercises:

1. **Name Your Emotions**:

When you notice strong emotions arising, take a moment to identify and label them. Use descriptive words such as "anxious," "frustrated," or "excited."

2. **Grounding Techniques**:

Engage in grounding exercises such as the 5-4-3-2-1 technique mentioned earlier. This technique involves naming five things you can see, four things you can touch, three things you can hear, two things you can smell, and one thing you can taste.

3. **Self-Compassion Meditation**:

   Practice self-compassion by offering kind and supportive words to yourself. Sit quietly and repeat phrases such as "May I be kind to myself," "May I be patient," and "May I accept myself as I am."

Benefits of Emotional Regulation Exercises:

- **Improved Relationships**: Better emotional regulation leads to more stable and constructive interactions with others, fostering healthier relationships.

- **Greater Resilience**: Regular practice builds emotional resilience, enabling individuals to bounce back from setbacks and challenges more effectively.

Applications:

- **Stressful Situations**: Use these techniques during stressful moments to calm your mind and respond to challenges with clarity and composure.

- **Therapeutic Settings**: Emotional regulation exercises are valuable tools in therapy for individuals working on managing anxiety, depression, trauma, or other emotional difficulties.

By integrating these emotional regulation exercises into your life, you can cultivate greater self-awareness, emotional balance, and resilience in navigating the complexities of emotions and daily life.

Leg Shaking

Leg shaking is a simple yet effective technique for releasing physical tension, promoting relaxation, and restoring balance to the body. This practice is especially beneficial for reducing stress, anxiety, and nervous energy accumulated throughout the day.

How to Practice Leg Shaking:

1. **Find a Comfortable Seated Position**:

   Sit comfortably in a chair with your feet flat on the ground and your spine upright. Ensure your legs are uncrossed and your arms are relaxed.

2. **Begin the Shaking Motion**:

   Start by lifting one leg slightly off the ground and begin shaking it gently from the hip down to the foot. Allow the shaking motion to be natural and rhythmic.

3. **Focus on Relaxation**:

   As you shake your leg, focus on releasing any tension or stiffness in the muscles. Let go of any stress or anxiety you may be holding in your body.

Benefits of Leg Shaking:

- **Tension Release**: Leg shaking helps release tension stored in the muscles, particularly in the lower body and legs.

- **Stress Reduction**: This practice promotes relaxation and reduces stress by activating the body's natural relaxation response.

Applications:

- **Before Bed**: Practice leg shaking before bedtime to unwind and prepare your body for restful sleep.

- **During Breaks**: Use leg shaking during breaks at work or study to refresh your mind and body.

Leg shaking is a simple yet powerful technique that anyone can practice to promote relaxation, release tension, and restore balance to the body.

Butterfly Pose

Butterfly pose, also known as Bound Angle Pose or Baddha Konasana in yoga, is a seated posture that stretches the inner thighs, groins, and knees while helping to calm the mind and promote relaxation.

How to Practice Butterfly Pose:

1. **Bring the Soles of Your Feet Together**:

   Bend your knees and bring the soles of your feet together, allowing your knees to drop out to the sides.

2. **Hold Your Feet with Your Hands**:

   Hold your feet or ankles with your hands. You can interlace your fingers around your toes or hold your ankles, depending on your flexibility.

3. **Sit Tall and Lengthen Your Spine**:

   Inhale and lengthen your spine upward. Imagine lifting through the crown of your head while keeping your shoulders relaxed and away from your ears.

4. **Open Your Hips**:

   Press your knees gently down toward the floor. Avoid forcing them; instead, let gravity and your breath gradually open your hips and inner thighs.

Benefits of Butterfly Pose:

- **Hip Opening**: Butterfly pose stretches and opens the hip flexors, groin, and inner thighs, improving flexibility and mobility in the hips.

- **Relaxation**: This pose promotes relaxation and helps calm the mind by encouraging deep, mindful breathing.

Applications:

- **Preparation for Meditation**: Use butterfly pose as a preparatory posture for meditation to create openness and ease in the hips.

- **During Work Breaks**: Practice this pose during breaks at work or study to release tension and refresh your mind.

- **Before Bed**: Incorporate butterfly pose into your bedtime routine to unwind and relax tight muscles before sleep.

Butterfly pose is a gentle yet effective posture for opening the hips, promoting relaxation, and fostering a sense of calm and well-being.

CHAPTER 5

EXERCISE FOR PAIN RELIEF

Slow Neck Rotations

Slow neck rotations are a gentle exercise that helps relieve tension and stiffness in the neck muscles while improving mobility and flexibility.

How to Practice Slow Neck Rotations:

1. **Relax Your Shoulders**:

   Keep your shoulders relaxed and away from your ears throughout the exercise.

2. **Slowly Rotate Your Neck**:

   Begin by gently dropping your chin towards your chest to stretch the back of your neck.

   Slowly rotate your head to the right, bringing your right ear towards your right shoulder.

   Hold this position for a few seconds, feeling a gentle stretch along the left side of your neck.

   Return your head to the center position.

3. **Repeat Several Times**:

   Continue to rotate your neck slowly from side to side, moving with awareness and focusing on the gentle stretch in each direction.

   Aim for 5-10 repetitions on each side, or as feels comfortable for you.

Benefits of Slow Neck Rotations:

- **Tension Relief**: Helps alleviate tension and tightness in the neck muscles, reducing discomfort and stiffness.

- **Improved Mobility**: Increases flexibility and range of motion in the neck, promoting ease of movement.

- **Mind-Body Connection**: Enhances awareness of posture and body alignment, fostering a greater sense of relaxation and well-being.

Applications:

- **Daily Practice**: Incorporate slow neck rotations into your daily routine to maintain neck health and prevent stiffness.

- **During Breaks**: Use this exercise during work breaks or long periods of sitting to refresh and relax the neck muscles.

- **Before Bed**: Practice slow neck rotations before bedtime to release tension and promote relaxation for a more restful sleep.

Slow neck rotations are a simple yet effective exercise that can be done almost anywhere to relieve neck tension and improve mobility.

Lateral Neck Tilts with Manual Resistance

Lateral neck tilts with manual resistance is an exercise designed to strengthen and stretch the muscles on the sides of the neck, promoting stability and flexibility in this area.

How to Practice Lateral Neck Tilts with Manual Resistance:

1. **Find a Comfortable Seated or Standing Position**:

   Sit upright in a chair with your spine straight, or stand with your feet hip-width apart and shoulders relaxed.

2. **Place Your Hand on Your Temple**:

   Start by placing your right hand gently on the right side of your head, just above your temple.

3. **Tilt Your Head to the Side**:

Inhale deeply, and as you exhale, gently tilt your head to the right side against the resistance of your hand.

Your hand should provide gentle resistance, but avoid pushing or pulling too hard.

4. **Hold the Stretch**:

Hold the tilted position for 5-10 seconds, feeling a stretch along the left side of your neck.

Maintain a steady breath throughout the stretch, inhaling and exhaling deeply.

Benefits of Lateral Neck Tilts with Manual Resistance:

- **Strengthens Neck Muscles**: Provides resistance to the neck muscles, enhancing their strength and endurance.
- **Increases Flexibility**: Improves flexibility and range of motion in the neck, reducing stiffness and discomfort.

Applications:

- **Neck Strengthening**: Incorporate this exercise into your routine to strengthen the neck muscles, which can help prevent strain and injury.
- **Relief from Tension**: Use it during breaks or after long periods of sitting to relieve tension and improve circulation in the neck area.

Lateral neck tilts with manual resistance are an effective way to strengthen and stretch the neck muscles while promoting stability and flexibility.

Deep Breathing in Child's Pose

Deep breathing in Child's Pose combines the benefits of a gentle yoga posture with diaphragmatic breathing, promoting relaxation, stress relief, and a sense of grounding.

How to Practice Deep Breathing in Child's Pose:

1. **Start in Child's Pose**:

   Begin on your hands and knees on a yoga mat or soft surface. Sit back on your heels and lower your forehead to the mat.

   Extend your arms forward with palms resting on the mat or by your sides, whichever is more comfortable.

2. **Settle into the Pose**:

   Take a moment to settle into the posture. Allow your hips to sink towards your heels and your spine to lengthen.

3. **Begin Deep Breathing**:

   Inhale deeply through your nose, expanding your belly as you fill your lungs with air. Feel your lower back and sides expand with each breath.

   Exhale slowly and completely through your nose or mouth, allowing your chest and belly to relax and deflate.

4. **Focus on the Breath**:

   Continue deep breathing in a slow and controlled manner. Let each inhalation be a conscious, calming breath, and each exhalation a release of tension.

Benefits of Deep Breathing in Child's Pose:

- **Stress Relief**: Deep breathing combined with the gentle stretch of Child's Pose helps release physical and mental tension.

- **Grounding**: Encourages a sense of grounding and inner calm, fostering a connection between mind and body.

Applications:

- **Daily Practice**: Incorporate deep breathing in Child's Pose into your daily routine as a relaxation technique and stress management tool.

- **Before Sleep**: Practice before bedtime to unwind and prepare your body and mind for restful sleep.

- **During Breaks**: Use it during work breaks or moments of overwhelm to reset and regain focus.

Deep breathing in Child's Pose offers a simple yet powerful way to relax, relieve stress, and cultivate a sense of peace and balance in your daily life.

Myofascial Massage with Tennis Ball under the Neck

Myofascial massage using a tennis ball under the neck is an effective self-care technique for releasing tension in the muscles and fascia of the neck and upper back.

How to Perform Myofascial Massage with Tennis Ball under the Neck:

1. **Preparation**:

   Find a quiet and comfortable space where you can lie down on your back, such as a yoga mat or carpeted floor.

   Have a tennis ball or a similar sized ball ready for the massage.

2. **Positioning**:

   Lie down on your back and place the tennis ball under your neck, targeting the area where you feel tension or discomfort.

   Adjust the position of the ball to ensure it is placed under a specific spot where you want to focus the massage.

3. **Apply Gentle Pressure**:

   Once the tennis ball is in position, relax your body and allow your weight to sink into the ball.

Apply gentle pressure by rolling the ball slightly side to side or up and down to find tight or tender spots.

Benefits of Myofascial Massage with Tennis Ball under the Neck:

- **Improved Circulation**: Stimulates blood flow to the targeted areas, promoting healing and relaxation.

- **Stress Reduction**: Helps alleviate stress and promote a sense of calm and relaxation.

Applications:

- **Self-Care Routine**: Incorporate this technique into your self-care routine to relieve neck and upper back tension, especially after long hours of sitting or physical activity.

- **Before Sleep**: Practice before bedtime to relax your muscles and improve sleep quality.

- **During Breaks**: Use it during work breaks or study breaks to refresh and release tension.

Myofascial massage with a tennis ball under the neck offers a simple yet effective way to alleviate tension, promote relaxation, and enhance overall well-being.

Controlled Breathing in Cat-Cow Pose

Controlled breathing in Cat-Cow Pose combines the benefits of mindful breathing with gentle spinal movement, promoting relaxation, breath awareness, and flexibility.

How to Practice Controlled Breathing in Cat-Cow Pose:

1. **Starting Position**:

   Begin on your hands and knees in a tabletop position on a yoga mat or soft surface. Ensure your wrists are directly under your shoulders and your knees under your hips.

2. **Cat Pose (Exhalation)**:

Inhale deeply through your nose, expanding your belly as you arch your back towards the ceiling.

Tuck your chin towards your chest and draw your belly button towards your spine, rounding your back like a cat stretching.

Exhale fully and completely through your mouth or nose as you hold this position.

3. **Cow Pose (Inhalation)**:

On your next inhalation, slowly lift your head and tailbone towards the ceiling.

Allow your belly to drop towards the floor, arching your back in the opposite direction.

Lift your gaze slightly towards the ceiling, keeping your shoulders away from your ears.

4. **Flow Between Poses**:

Flow smoothly between Cat and Cow Poses with each breath cycle, moving at a pace that feels comfortable and fluid for you.

Continue the controlled breathing and gentle spinal movement for 5-10 rounds, or as long as feels soothing and beneficial.

Benefits of Controlled Breathing in Cat-Cow Pose:

- **Breath Awareness**: Enhances awareness of the breath, promoting mindfulness and relaxation.

- **Spinal Mobility**: Improves flexibility and mobility in the spine, reducing stiffness and enhancing posture.

- **Stress Reduction**: Calms the mind and nervous system, reducing stress and promoting a sense of inner peace.

Applications:

- **Daily Practice**: Include controlled breathing in Cat-Cow Pose as part of your daily yoga or mindfulness routine to promote overall well-being.

- **Before Meditation**: Use it as a preparatory practice before meditation to center the mind and body.

- **During Stressful Times**: Practice during moments of stress or tension to help restore balance and calm.

Controlled breathing in Cat-Cow Pose offers a gentle yet effective way to integrate breath awareness with spinal movement, fostering relaxation, flexibility, and mindfulness in your daily life.

Circular Shoulder Movements to Relieve Tension

Circular shoulder movements are a simple and effective exercise to release tension in the shoulders, neck, and upper back, promoting relaxation and enhancing mobility.

How to Perform Circular Shoulder Movements:

1. **Starting Position**:

   Stand or sit comfortably with your spine straight and shoulders relaxed. You can also perform this exercise while standing or sitting on a chair with a straight back.

2. **Shoulder Roll Backwards**:

   Begin by inhaling deeply as you lift your shoulders towards your ears, tensing the muscles slightly.

   Exhale slowly and roll your shoulders backward in a circular motion. Imagine drawing a circle with your shoulders, moving them away from your ears and down towards your back.

Continue the circular motion, feeling the stretch and release in your shoulder muscles.

3. **Complete Several Rotations**:

Perform 5-10 backward shoulder rotations in a slow and controlled manner.

Focus on the quality of the movement, allowing your breath to guide the flow of the circular motion.

4. **Shoulder Roll Forward**:

After completing backward rotations, reverse the movement.

Inhale deeply and lift your shoulders towards your ears.

Exhale slowly as you roll your shoulders forward in a circular motion, bringing them forward, down, and back up towards your ears.

Continue the forward circular motion for 5-10 rotations, maintaining a gentle and fluid movement.

Benefits of Circular Shoulder Movements:

- **Tension Relief**: Releases tension and tightness in the shoulders, neck, and upper back.
- **Improved Mobility**: Enhances flexibility and mobility in the shoulder joints, reducing stiffness and improving range of motion.
- **Stress Reduction**: Promotes relaxation and calms the nervous system, reducing overall stress and tension.

Applications:

- **Daily Practice**: Include circular shoulder movements as part of your daily routine to maintain shoulder health and prevent stiffness.

- **Before Physical Activity**: Warm up with shoulder rotations before engaging in physical activities or exercises that involve the upper body.

- **During Breaks**: Use it during work breaks or study breaks to relieve muscle tension and refresh your mind.

Circular shoulder movements are a versatile exercise that can be performed anywhere and anytime to relieve tension, improve mobility, and promote relaxation in your shoulders and upper body.

PILATES EXERCISES FOR LOWER BACK PAIN REDUCTION
Psoas Release Exercise

The psoas muscle, located deep within the core, plays a crucial role in stabilizing the spine and supporting movement. When tight or tense, it can contribute to lower back pain, hip discomfort, and even affect overall posture. This chapter explores a gentle and effective psoas release exercise aimed at reducing tension and enhancing mobility.

Benefits of Supine Knee-to-Chest Stretch:

- **Relieves Lower Back Pain**: By stretching the psoas muscle, this exercise helps alleviate tension and pain in the lower back.

- **Improves Hip Flexibility**: Enhances flexibility in the hip joints, promoting better range of motion.

- **Promotes Relaxation**: Helps relax the muscles of the lower back and hips, reducing overall tension and promoting a sense of well-being.

How to Perform the Supine Knee-to-Chest Stretch:

1. **Starting Position**:

   Lie down on your back on a yoga mat or comfortable surface.

Extend your legs straight and relax your arms by your sides.

2. **Engage Mindfully**:

Take a few deep breaths to relax your body and focus your mind on the exercise.

Bring awareness to the area of your lower back and hips.

3. **Performing the Stretch**:

Bend your right knee and bring it towards your chest, using both hands to gently pull your knee closer to your body.

Hold your right knee with your hands clasped just below the kneecap or behind the thigh, depending on your flexibility.

Keep your left leg extended on the mat or bend it slightly for comfort.

Tips for Effective Stretching:

- **Gentle Movement**: Perform the stretch with slow, controlled movements to avoid any sudden or jerky motions.

- **Listen to Your Body**: If you feel discomfort or pain, adjust the intensity or position of the stretch accordingly.

- **Regular Practice**: Incorporate this stretch into your daily routine to maintain flexibility and reduce tension in the psoas muscle over time.

Precautions:

- **Avoid Overstretching**: Stretch only to the point of mild tension, never to the point of pain.

- **Consultation**: If you have existing lower back issues or medical concerns, consult with a healthcare professional before starting this or any exercise program.

The supine knee-to-chest stretch is an excellent exercise for releasing tension in the psoas muscle and promoting flexibility in the lower back and hips.

Self-Massage

Self-massage is a valuable technique for easing muscle tension, promoting relaxation, and enhancing overall well-being. This chapter explores various self-massage techniques that you can perform on yourself to release tight muscles and reduce stress.

Benefits of Self-Massage:

- **Muscle Relaxation**: Helps to release tension in specific muscles, promoting relaxation and reducing stiffness.

- **Improved Circulation**: Enhances blood flow to the massaged area, aiding in nutrient delivery and waste removal.

- **Pain Relief**: Alleviates discomfort caused by muscle tightness, knots, or trigger points.

Tips for Effective Self-Massage:

- **Use Gentle Pressure**: Start with light pressure and gradually increase as needed, avoiding discomfort or pain.

- **Focus on Breathing**: Take slow, deep breaths as you massage to enhance relaxation and release tension.

- **Repeat Regularly**: Incorporate self-massage into your daily routine or as needed to maintain muscle health and reduce stress levels.

Precautions:

- **Avoid Injured Areas**: Do not massage directly over areas of acute injury, inflammation, or open wounds.

- **Consultation**: If you have chronic pain or medical conditions, consult with a healthcare professional before performing self-massage techniques.

Self-massage is a simple yet effective way to relax muscles, alleviate tension, and promote overall well-being.

Dear Reader,

Thank you for taking the time to read the first chapter of "Somatic Exercises for Beginners Overcome Stress, Chronic Pain, and Anxiety with 60+ Proven Techniques – a 28-Day Journey to Mind-Body Connection in 10 Minutes a Day | Includes Guided Video Tutorials" Your journey towards better health is important to us, and we hope that the insights provided here have been helpful and inspiring.

Your feedback is invaluable to us. It helps us understand what works well and what can be improved, ensuring that we can provide the best possible content to support you and others on similar paths. By sharing your thoughts, you not only help us improve but also assist other readers in finding the right resources for their needs.

How You Can Share Your Review on Amazon.com:

- Go to the Amazon page where you found my book.
- Navigate to the 'Customer Reviews' section.
- Click on 'Write a customer review' to share your valuable insights.

Instant QR Code Access: Simply scan the QR code below with your smartphone to be directed to the Amazon review section.

CHAPTER 6

EXERCISE FOR OVERCOMING TRAUMA

Trauma Release Exercises

Trauma release exercises (TRE) are designed to help individuals release deeply-held tension and stress stored in the body as a result of traumatic experiences. These exercises promote a natural shaking or trembling response, which aids in the discharge of muscular tension and emotional stress. This chapter explores the principles behind TRE and provides an introduction to some basic exercises.

Principles of Trauma Release Exercises

1. Neurogenic Tremors:

- TRE leverages neurogenic tremors, which are involuntary shaking or trembling movements that originate from the body's nervous system.

- These tremors are believed to be a natural, physiological response that helps the body release stored tension and restore a sense of equilibrium.

2. Gentle Activation:

- The exercises gently activate the body's tremor mechanism through specific movements and postures designed to induce tremors.

- Participants are encouraged to allow these tremors to occur naturally without trying to control or suppress them.

3. Self-Regulation:

- TRE emphasizes self-regulation, allowing individuals to manage their own experience and pace of tremor release.

- Participants are guided to listen to their bodies and respect their limits during the process.

Basic Trauma Release Exercises

1. Legs-Up-the-Wall Position:

- Lie on your back with your buttocks close to a wall and extend your legs vertically up the wall.

- Keep your arms relaxed by your sides, palms facing up.

- Focus on deep, diaphragmatic breathing and allow any natural tremors to arise in your legs and hips.

2. Bridge Position:

- Lie on your back with your knees bent and feet flat on the floor, hip-width apart.

- Slowly lift your hips towards the ceiling, creating a bridge with your body.

- Support your lower back with your hands or keep arms flat on the floor. Allow any tremors to release through your legs and core.

Benefits of Trauma Release Exercises

- **Tension Release**: Promotes the release of muscular tension and chronic holding patterns in the body.

- **Stress Reduction**: Helps to reduce stress hormones like cortisol and promotes a sense of relaxation.

- **Emotional Healing**: Facilitates the release of emotional stress and trauma stored in the body, supporting emotional resilience.

Precautions and Considerations

- **Professional Guidance**: It is advisable to learn TRE under the guidance of a certified TRE provider or therapist, especially if you have a history of trauma or significant emotional distress.

- **Listen to Your Body**: Pay attention to any discomfort or overwhelming emotions that may arise during the exercises. Take breaks as needed and seek support if necessary.

Trauma release exercises offer a unique approach to healing by harnessing the body's natural ability to release tension and trauma stored in muscles. By practicing these exercises mindfully and with proper guidance, individuals can experience relief from chronic stress, enhanced emotional well-being, and a greater sense of resilience in their daily lives.

Pendulation Movements

Pendulation movements are a core concept in somatic experiencing, a therapeutic approach developed by Dr. Peter Levine to address trauma. These movements involve gently oscillating between states of tension and relaxation, helping to restore balance to the nervous system and facilitating the release of trauma-related stress.

Principles of Pendulation Movements

1. Alternating States:

- Pendulation involves moving back and forth between states of heightened sensation or tension and states of calm or relaxation.

- This process helps the nervous system to recalibrate and restore its natural rhythm.

2. Gradual Exposure:

- The movements are designed to gently expose the body and mind to sensations associated with both activation and relaxation.

- This gradual exposure helps to build resilience and tolerance to stress, reducing the impact of traumatic memories.

Practicing Pendulation Movements

1. Sensing Tension and Relaxation:

- Begin by finding a comfortable seated or lying position in a quiet space.

- Close your eyes and take a few deep breaths, bringing your attention to your body.

- Notice any areas of tension or discomfort, and observe the sensations without judgment.

2. Focusing on Tension:

- Once you have identified an area of tension, focus your attention on it.

- Observe the sensations in this area, such as tightness, heat, or pressure.

- Stay with these sensations for a few moments, allowing yourself to fully experience them.

3. Shifting to Relaxation:

- After a few moments, shift your attention to an area of your body that feels calm or relaxed.

- Notice the sensations of relaxation, such as softness, warmth, or ease.

- Allow yourself to fully experience these sensations, letting them spread throughout your body.

4. Moving Back and Forth:

- Gently move your attention back to the area of tension, and then back to the area of relaxation.

- Continue to oscillate between these two states, spending a few moments in each.

- Notice how the sensations change and evolve with each movement.

Benefits of Pendulation Movements

- **Nervous System Regulation**: Helps to restore balance to the nervous system, reducing symptoms of hyperarousal and hypoarousal.

- **Trauma Release**: Facilitates the release of stored tension and stress associated with traumatic experiences.

- **Emotional Resilience**: Builds resilience and tolerance to stress, enhancing emotional well-being and stability.

Tips for Effective Pendulation Practice

- **Start Slowly**: Begin with short sessions and gradually increase the duration as you become more comfortable with the practice.

- **Stay Present**: Use mindful awareness to stay present and grounded during the movements. If you feel overwhelmed, take a break and return when you feel ready.

- **Seek Support**: If you have a history of trauma or significant emotional distress, consider practicing pendulation under the guidance of a trained therapist.

Pendulation movements are a powerful tool for balancing the nervous system and promoting the release of trauma-related tension and stress.

Grounding and Centering Exercises

Grounding and centering exercises are essential techniques in somatic experiencing and trauma recovery. These exercises help you reconnect with your body, stabilize your emotions, and anchor yourself in the present moment.

Benefits of Grounding and Centering Exercises

- **Emotional Stability**: Helps to stabilize emotions and reduce anxiety by bringing you back to the present moment.

- **Increased Awareness**: Enhances your ability to notice and manage bodily sensations and emotional responses.

- **Enhanced Resilience**: Builds resilience by providing tools to manage stress and recover more quickly from emotional disturbances.

Tips for Effective Practice

- **Regular Practice**: Incorporate grounding and centering exercises into your daily routine, even when you're not feeling stressed. This helps to build a strong foundation for emotional regulation.

- **Stay Patient**: Be patient with yourself as you learn these techniques. It may take time to feel the full benefits, but regular practice will lead to improvement.

- **Seek Support**: If you struggle with grounding or centering, consider seeking guidance from a therapist or somatic experiencing practitioner.

Grounding and centering exercises are powerful tools for managing stress, reducing anxiety, and enhancing emotional resilience.

Body-Mind Connection Exercises

The body-mind connection is a powerful concept that emphasizes the interdependence of physical and mental health.

Benefits of Body-Mind Connection Exercises

- **Reduces Stress**: Helps alleviate physical and mental stress by promoting relaxation.

- **Enhances Emotional Resilience**: Strengthens your ability to cope with emotional challenges.

- **Improves Self-Awareness**: Fosters a deeper understanding of the connection between your body and emotions.

- **Promotes Physical Health**: Supports overall physical well-being through mindful movement.

Practicing Body-Mind Connection Exercises

Body-mind connection exercises provide a holistic approach to enhancing emotional resilience, reducing stress, and promoting overall well-being.

Tai Chi Movements

At its core, Tai Chi emphasizes the smooth flow of energy, or "qi," throughout the body. The movements are designed to cultivate this energy, promoting physical health and emotional stability. Tai Chi is practiced in a sequence of postures or forms, each flowing seamlessly into the next. This continuous flow helps improve coordination, strength, and mindfulness.

Benefits of Tai Chi Movements

- **Enhances Balance and Coordination**: Regular practice improves physical stability and coordination.

- **Reduces Stress and Anxiety**: The meditative nature of Tai Chi helps calm the mind and reduce stress.

- **Promotes Flexibility and Strength**: Slow, controlled movements enhance muscle strength and flexibility.

Practicing Tai Chi Movements

1. Preparation (Wu Ji)

The preparation posture sets the stage for your Tai Chi practice, helping you center your mind and body.

- **How to Practice**:

    Stand with your feet shoulder-width apart, knees slightly bent.

    Let your arms hang naturally by your sides.

    Close your eyes or keep them softly focused ahead.

    Take a few deep breaths, feeling your connection to the ground.

    Visualize your body as a stable, rooted tree.

2. Commencement (Qi Shi)

The commencement posture initiates the flow of energy and prepares you for the following movements.

- **How to Practice**:

    From the preparation posture, slowly raise your arms in front of you to shoulder height, palms facing down.

    As you inhale, let your arms float up, feeling lightness and openness in your chest.

    As you exhale, slowly lower your arms back to your sides, maintaining a sense of calm and relaxation.

3. Parting the Wild Horse's Mane (Ye Ma Fen Zong)

This movement mimics the graceful motion of a horse's mane, enhancing balance and coordination.

- **How to Practice**:

    Step your left foot to the side, shifting your weight onto it.

    Simultaneously, bring your left hand in front of your chest, palm facing inward, while your right hand moves to your side, palm facing down.

Shift your weight to your right foot and repeat the motion on the other side, stepping your right foot out and switching hand positions.

Continue the sequence, focusing on smooth, flowing transitions and coordinated movement.

Incorporating Tai Chi into your daily routine can yield significant benefits for both physical and mental health. Start with a few minutes each day, gradually increasing the duration as you become more comfortable with the movements. Practice in a quiet, open space where you can move freely and focus on your breath and body.

Spinal Twists

The spine is a central axis of the body, housing the spinal cord and supporting overall posture and movement.

Benefits of Spinal Twists

- **Improves Spinal Flexibility**: Regular practice of spinal twists enhances the flexibility and range of motion of the spine.

- **Relieves Tension**: Twisting motions help release built-up tension in the back, shoulders, and neck.

- **Enhances Circulation**: These movements promote blood flow to the spinal muscles and surrounding tissues, aiding in nutrient delivery and waste removal.

Performing Spinal Twists

Seated Spinal Twist (Ardha Matsyendrasana)

The seated spinal twist is a foundational twist that gently stretches the spine and massages the abdominal organs.

- **How to Practice:**

Sit on the floor with your legs extended in front of you.

Bend your right knee and place your right foot on the outside of your left thigh.

Bend your left knee and bring your left foot near your right hip, or keep your left leg extended if this is uncomfortable.

Supine Spinal Twist (Supta Matsyendrasana)

The supine spinal twist is a gentle, restorative twist performed lying down, ideal for releasing lower back tension.

- **How to Practice**:

Lie on your back with your legs extended.

Bend your right knee and bring it toward your chest.

Extend your right arm out to the side at shoulder height, palm facing up.

Use your left hand to guide your right knee across your body toward the left side.

Keep both shoulders grounded and turn your head to the right.

Hold the twist for several breaths, feeling the stretch along your spine and the release of tension.

Return to the starting position and repeat on the opposite side.

Standing Spinal Twist

The standing spinal twist is a dynamic twist that can be performed anywhere, promoting spinal mobility and energy flow.

- **How to Practice**:

Stand with your feet hip-width apart and your arms by your sides.

Inhale, lengthen your spine, and lift your arms to shoulder height.

Exhale, and gently twist your torso to the right, allowing your arms to swing naturally.

Inhale, return to center, and exhale, twist to the left.

Continue alternating sides in a smooth, rhythmic motion, focusing on your breath and the gentle twisting of your spine.

Integrating Spinal Twists into Daily Routine

Incorporating spinal twists into your daily routine can have lasting benefits for your physical and emotional health. Start with a few minutes each day, practicing the twists that feel most comfortable and beneficial for your body. These exercises can be performed in the morning to energize your spine and throughout the day to release tension and promote relaxation.

Pelvic Tilts

Pelvic tilts are a fundamental exercise in somatic practices that help strengthen the lower back and abdominal muscles, improve pelvic alignment, and reduce pain. This exercise is gentle and can be performed by individuals of all fitness levels. In this chapter, we will explore the benefits of pelvic tilts, provide detailed instructions for performing the exercise, and offer tips for integrating pelvic tilts into your daily routine.

Benefits of Pelvic Tilts

- **Strengthens Core Muscles**: Engaging the abdominal and lower back muscles during pelvic tilts helps build a strong core, providing better support for the spine.

- **Improves Pelvic Alignment**: Regular practice of pelvic tilts promotes proper alignment of the pelvis, reducing strain on the lower back.

- **Reduces Back Pain**: By mobilizing the pelvis and strengthening the supporting muscles, pelvic tilts can alleviate lower back pain and discomfort.

- **Enhances Body Awareness**: Performing pelvic tilts with mindfulness helps increase awareness of pelvic positioning and movement, contributing to better overall posture.

- **Supports Spinal Health**: Gentle mobilization of the pelvis aids in maintaining spinal flexibility and health.

Performing Pelvic Tilts

Supine Pelvic Tilts

The supine pelvic tilt is a basic version of the exercise, performed while lying on your back. It is a gentle and effective way to engage the core muscles and mobilize the pelvis.

- **How to Practice**:

  Lie on your back with your knees bent and feet flat on the floor, hip-width apart.

  Place your arms by your sides, palms facing down.

  Inhale deeply, allowing your lower back to arch slightly away from the floor.

  Exhale, gently press your lower back into the floor by tilting your pelvis upward, engaging your abdominal muscles.

  Hold the tilt for a moment, then inhale and return to the starting position with a slight arch in your lower back.

  Repeat the movement for 10-15 repetitions, focusing on a smooth and controlled motion.

Standing Pelvic Tilts

Standing pelvic tilts are a more advanced version of the exercise, performed in an upright position. This variation helps improve pelvic alignment and core strength while standing.

- **How to Practice**:

  Stand with your feet hip-width apart and your knees slightly bent.

  Place your hands on your hips, with your fingers resting on your lower abdomen and your thumbs on your lower back.

  Inhale, allowing your pelvis to tilt slightly forward, creating a gentle arch in your lower back.

  Exhale, gently tilt your pelvis backward, flattening your lower back and engaging your abdominal muscles.

  Hold the tilt for a moment, then inhale and return to the starting position.

Tips for Integrating Pelvic Tilts into Your Routine

Incorporating pelvic tilts into your daily routine can have significant benefits for your spinal and pelvic health. Here are some tips to help you integrate this exercise effectively:

- **Consistency**: Practice pelvic tilts daily to build strength and improve pelvic alignment.

- **Mindfulness**: Perform the exercise with awareness, focusing on the movement and engagement of your core muscles.

- **Breath**: Coordinate your breath with the movement, inhaling as you arch your lower back and exhaling as you tilt your pelvis.

- **Warm-Up**: Include pelvic tilts as part of your warm-up routine before engaging in other physical activities or exercises.

Pelvic tilts are a simple yet powerful exercise for improving core strength, pelvic alignment, and reducing lower back pain.

CHAPTER 7

EXERCISE FOR POSTURE AND FLEXIBILITY

Dynamic Stretching

Dynamic stretching is an effective method for preparing the body for physical activity by increasing blood flow, enhancing muscular performance, and improving flexibility.

Importance of Dynamic Stretching

Dynamic stretching serves multiple purposes in preparing the body for physical activity. By engaging in these movements, you can effectively prepare your muscles and joints for the demands of exercise, reduce stiffness, and enhance overall performance. Here are some key benefits:

- **Increased Blood Flow**: Dynamic movements stimulate circulation, delivering more oxygen and nutrients to muscles, which can enhance performance and reduce the risk of injury.

- **Improved Flexibility**: Regular practice of dynamic stretching increases the flexibility of muscles and joints, making it easier to perform various physical activities.

- **Enhanced Muscular Performance**: Dynamic stretching activates muscles and enhances neuromuscular coordination, which can lead to better performance in sports and exercise.

- **Injury Prevention**: By warming up the muscles and joints, dynamic stretching reduces the likelihood of strains and other injuries during physical activity.

- **Mental Preparation**: Engaging in dynamic stretching helps to mentally prepare for exercise, improving focus and readiness.

Performing Dynamic Stretching Exercises

Dynamic stretching exercises involve fluid movements that mimic the activities or sports you are about to perform. Here are some effective dynamic stretching exercises to include in your warm-up routine:

Leg Swings

Leg swings are excellent for loosening up the hip joints and preparing the legs for running or other lower-body activities.

- **How to Practice**:

    Stand next to a wall or hold onto a stable surface for balance.

    Swing your right leg forward and backward in a controlled manner, gradually increasing the range of motion.

    Perform 10-15 swings, then switch to the left leg and repeat.

    Next, swing your right leg side to side, crossing in front of your body and then out to the side.

    Perform 10-15 swings, then switch to the left leg and repeat.

Arm Circles

Arm circles help to warm up the shoulder joints and upper body muscles, making them ideal for activities that involve the arms.

- **How to Practice**:

    Stand with your feet shoulder-width apart and extend your arms out to the sides at shoulder height.

    Make small circles with your arms, gradually increasing the size of the circles.

    Perform 10-15 circles in a forward direction, then switch to backward circles.

    Repeat the movement, increasing the circle size as you go.

Walking Lunges

Walking lunges are effective for warming up the legs, hips, and glutes, and improving balance and coordination.

- **How to Practice**:

    Stand with your feet hip-width apart.

    Step forward with your right leg, lowering into a lunge position with both knees bent at 90 degrees.

    Push off with your left foot and bring it forward to step into the next lunge.

    Continue moving forward in a lunge walk for 10-15 steps on each leg.

    Keep your torso upright and engage your core throughout the movement.

Torso Twists

Torso twists help to loosen up the spine and improve rotational mobility, which is beneficial for various sports and activities.

- **How to Practice**:

    Stand with your feet shoulder-width apart and your knees slightly bent.

    Place your hands on your hips or extend your arms out to the sides.

    Rotate your torso to the right, then to the left, allowing your hips to follow the movement.

    Perform 10-15 twists on each side, maintaining a controlled and fluid motion.

Tips for Incorporating Dynamic Stretching

To maximize the benefits of dynamic stretching, it is important to integrate these exercises into your warm-up routine effectively. Here are some tips:

- **Warm-Up First**: Start with a light aerobic activity, such as jogging or brisk walking, to increase your heart rate and warm up your muscles before performing dynamic stretches.

- **Focus on Major Muscle Groups**: Target the major muscle groups that will be engaged in your workout or sport. This ensures that your body is adequately prepared for the activity.

- **Maintain Control**: Perform each movement in a controlled manner, avoiding jerky or rapid motions that could lead to injury.

- **Gradually Increase Intensity**: Begin with smaller movements and gradually increase the range and intensity as your muscles warm up.

- **Consistency**: Make dynamic stretching a regular part of your pre-exercise routine to consistently improve flexibility, performance, and reduce injury risk.

Dynamic stretching is an essential component of an effective warm-up routine, offering numerous benefits for flexibility, performance, and injury prevention. By incorporating dynamic stretching exercises, such as leg swings, arm circles, walking lunges, and torso twists, you can prepare your body for physical activity and enhance your overall fitness experience.

Fluid and Circular Movements

Fluid and circular movements are integral to somatic practices, focusing on gentle, continuous motions that promote flexibility, coordination, and relaxation.

The Benefits of Fluid and Circular Movements

Fluid and circular movements offer numerous benefits that contribute to overall physical and mental health. These exercises help to:

- **Enhance Flexibility**: Gentle, flowing motions stretch and lengthen muscles, improving overall flexibility.

- **Improve Joint Mobility**: Circular movements lubricate joints, increasing their range of motion and reducing stiffness.

- **Promote Relaxation**: The rhythmic nature of these exercises helps to calm the nervous system, reducing stress and anxiety.

- **Increase Body Awareness**: Engaging in fluid movements enhances proprioception, or the sense of where your body is in space, leading to better coordination and balance.

- **Facilitate Tension Release**: Continuous, gentle movements can help release physical and emotional tension stored in the body.

Performing Fluid and Circular Movements

Incorporating fluid and circular movements into your exercise routine can be simple and enjoyable. Here are some exercises to get you started:

Arm Circles

Arm circles are a fundamental fluid movement that helps to warm up the shoulders and improve upper body flexibility.

- **How to Practice**:

  Stand with your feet shoulder-width apart and arms extended out to the sides at shoulder height.

  Begin making small circles with your arms, gradually increasing the size of the circles.

  Perform 10-15 circles in a forward direction, then switch to backward circles.

Hip Circles

Hip circles are excellent for loosening up the hips and lower back, enhancing mobility in these areas.

- **How to Practice**:

    Stand with your feet shoulder-width apart and hands on your hips.

    Begin moving your hips in a circular motion, starting with small circles and gradually making them larger.

    Perform 10-15 circles in one direction, then switch to the opposite direction.

    Keep your knees slightly bent and your movements fluid and continuous.

Fluid and circular movements are a gentle yet effective way to enhance flexibility, improve joint mobility, and promote overall relaxation and well-being.

Spinal Relaxation and Stretching Practices

Maintaining spinal health is crucial for overall mobility, posture, and reducing the risk of back pain. Incorporating relaxation techniques and specific stretches can help alleviate tension, improve flexibility, and promote spinal alignment.

Balance and Coordination Exercises

Improving balance and coordination is essential for enhancing stability, preventing falls, and optimizing overall physical performance. Incorporating specific exercises into your routine can help strengthen muscles, improve proprioception (awareness of body position), and enhance coordination skills. In this chapter, we explore effective exercises designed to enhance balance and coordination.

1. Single-Leg Stance

- **How to Practice**:

Stand tall with your feet hip-width apart.

Shift your weight onto one leg and lift the opposite foot off the ground.

Find a focal point to maintain balance and engage your core muscles.

Hold for 20-30 seconds, then switch legs.

Progress by extending the hold time or closing your eyes for an added challenge.

2. Heel-to-Toe Walk (Tandem Walk)

- **How to Practice**:

Stand with your feet in a straight line, placing the heel of one foot directly in front of the toes of the other foot.

Keep your arms relaxed by your sides or extended for balance.

Take slow and deliberate steps, placing each foot directly in front of the other.

Walk this way for 10-20 steps forward, then reverse direction.

3. Standing Balance Exercises

- **Tree Pose (Vrksasana)**:

Stand tall with your feet hip-width apart.

Shift your weight onto one foot and lift the opposite foot off the ground.

Place the sole of your lifted foot on the inner thigh or calf of the standing leg.

Bring your palms together in front of your chest or extend your arms overhead.

Hold for 20-30 seconds, then switch sides.

- **Flamingo Stand**:

Stand on one leg and lift the opposite foot slightly off the ground.

Hold onto a stable surface for balance if needed.

Extend your lifted leg backward and hold for 10-15 seconds.

Return to the starting position and repeat on the other side.

4. Coordination Exercises

- **Ball Toss and Catch**:

Stand facing a partner or a wall at a comfortable distance.

Toss a small ball gently back and forth, aiming for accuracy and smooth coordination.

Increase the speed or vary the height and angle of your tosses for added challenge.

5. Tai Chi or Qi Gong Movements

- **Tai Chi "Cloud Hands"**:

Begin in a standing position with feet shoulder-width apart and knees slightly bent.

Sweep your arms in a circular motion to one side while shifting your weight.

Repeat this flowing movement to the other side, coordinating with your breath.

Practice slowly and smoothly for 1-2 minutes to improve coordination and balance.

Tips for Balance and Coordination

- **Consistency**: Practice these exercises regularly to improve balance and coordination skills over time.

- **Safety First**: Use a stable surface or support when needed to prevent falls and injuries.

- **Progression**: Gradually increase the difficulty of exercises as your balance and coordination improve.

- **Mind-Body Connection**: Focus on your movements and maintain awareness of your body's position and alignment.

Incorporating balance and coordination exercises into your fitness routine can significantly enhance your stability, prevent falls, and improve overall physical performance. By practicing these exercises consistently and mindfully, you can strengthen muscles, enhance proprioception, and develop better coordination skills. Whether you're aiming to improve sports performance or maintain independence in daily activities, these exercises offer valuable benefits for your overall well-being. Remember to start gradually, listen to your body, and enjoy the process of enhancing your balance and coordination abilities.

Spinal Twists

Spinal twists are beneficial exercises that enhance spinal mobility, stretch muscles along the back, and promote overall flexibility. These exercises help alleviate tension, improve circulation, and maintain spinal health. Incorporate these gentle twists into your routine to enjoy their therapeutic benefits.

1. Seated Spinal Twist (Ardha Matsyendrasana)

- **How to Practice**:

  Sit on the floor with your legs extended straight in front of you.

  Bend your right knee and place your right foot flat on the floor outside your left thigh.

Keep your left leg extended or bend it and place your left foot outside your right hip.

Inhale and lengthen your spine, then exhale and twist your torso to the right, placing your left hand on your right knee and your right hand behind you for support.

Hold the twist for 30 seconds to 1 minute, breathing deeply.

Release the twist on an exhale and repeat on the opposite side.

2. Supine Spinal Twist (Supta Matsyendrasana)

- **How to Practice**:

Lie on your back with your legs extended.

Bend your knees and draw them towards your chest.

Extend your arms straight out to the sides at shoulder height.

Exhale and lower both knees to one side, keeping your shoulders grounded.

Turn your head to the opposite side of your knees.

Hold the twist for 30 seconds to 1 minute, breathing deeply into your belly.

Inhale to return your knees to center, then exhale and repeat on the other side.

3. Standing Spinal Twist

- **How to Practice**:

Stand with your feet hip-width apart.

Extend your arms straight out to the sides at shoulder height.

Inhale to lengthen your spine, then exhale and twist your torso to the right, bringing your left hand to your right shoulder and your right hand to the small of your back.

Hold the twist for 15-30 seconds, maintaining steady breathing.

Inhale to return to center, then exhale and repeat on the left side.

Tips for Spinal Twists

- **Warm-Up**: Always warm up your spine with gentle movements before performing deeper spinal twists.

- **Alignment**: Focus on maintaining length in your spine during twists to avoid compressing the vertebrae.

- **Breathing**: Coordinate your breath with the movement to deepen the stretch and enhance relaxation.

- **Mindfulness**: Be mindful of any discomfort or strain, and modify the twist as needed to suit your flexibility and comfort level.

Spinal twists are effective exercises for enhancing spinal mobility, relieving tension, and improving overall flexibility.

Rolling Down the Spine

1. **Starting Position**:

   Stand tall with your feet hip-width apart and arms relaxed by your sides.

   Take a moment to center yourself and bring awareness to your posture.

2. **Initiating the Movement**:

   Inhale deeply and engage your core muscles.

   Slowly begin to roll your chin towards your chest, allowing your head to lead the movement.

Continue to roll your spine down, one vertebra at a time, towards the floor.

3. **Midway Point**:

As you continue rolling down, allow your arms to hang freely towards the floor.

Keep your knees slightly bent to maintain a gentle stretch in your lower back.

4. **Repeat**:

Perform 5-10 repetitions of rolling down the spine, moving with your breath and focusing on releasing tension with each descent.

Tips for Rolling Down the Spine:

- **Controlled Movement**: Move slowly and mindfully, allowing each vertebra to articulate sequentially.

- **Alignment**: Maintain a neutral spine throughout the movement to avoid excessive rounding or arching.

- **Modification**: If standing is uncomfortable, perform this exercise seated on a chair or the floor with your legs extended.

Benefits of Rolling Down the Spine:

- **Spinal Mobilization**: Helps to improve flexibility and mobility of the spine.

- **Muscle Relaxation**: Releases tension in the back muscles, promoting relaxation.

- **Postural Awareness**: Enhances body awareness and posture by gently stretching and aligning the spine.

Incorporate rolling down the spine into your daily routine as a gentle exercise to promote spinal health, release tension, and improve overall flexibility. It's an effective way to maintain mobility and alleviate stiffness, particularly after long periods of sitting or standing.

Child's Pose

Child's Pose, known as Balasana in yoga, is a restful and grounding posture that stretches and relaxes the muscles of the back, hips, and thighs. It's often used in yoga practice as a resting pose or as a gentle stretch to release tension in the spine and promote relaxation. Here's how to perform Child's Pose:

Child's Pose (Balasana)

1. **Starting Position**:

   Begin on your hands and knees in a tabletop position (also known as "Cat-Cow" position).

   Ensure your wrists are directly under your shoulders and your knees are under your hips.

2. **Execution**:

   Take a deep breath in.

   As you exhale, slowly lower your hips back towards your heels.

   Keep your arms extended in front of you or relax them alongside your body, palms facing up.

   Allow your forehead to rest gently on the mat or the floor.

3. **Alignment**:

   Extend your spine long and keep your neck in a neutral position.

   If your forehead doesn't comfortably reach the ground, you can place a yoga block or a folded towel under your forehead for support.

Relax your shoulders away from your ears and soften any tension in your face and jaw.

4. **Modifications**:

For a wider stance, separate your knees slightly wider than hip-width apart to create more space for your torso between your thighs.

If you have knee discomfort, place a folded blanket or cushion between your thighs and calves for added support.

Benefits of Child's Pose:

- **Spinal Stretch**: Gentle stretch for the spine, relieving tension in the lower back.

- **Hip Opener**: Opens the hips and stretches the muscles of the hips and thighs.

- **Relaxation**: Promotes relaxation by encouraging deep breathing and calming the mind.

- **Stress Relief**: Relieves stress and fatigue, making it an excellent pose to practice during times of emotional strain or overwhelm.

Contraindications:

- Avoid Child's Pose if you have knee injuries or discomfort unless using additional support.

- If you have digestive issues, it may be more comfortable to keep your knees closer together to avoid pressure on the abdomen.

Child's Pose is a nurturing posture that offers physical and emotional benefits. It's a simple yet powerful way to restore your energy, find calmness, and gently stretch your body, making it suitable for practitioners of all levels and ages.

CHAPTER 8
THE 28-DAY SOMATIC CHALLENGE (BONUS CHAPTER)

A 28 Day-by-Day Guide to Transforming Your Body and Mind with 10 minutes per day (Bonus)

28-Day Somatic Training Program

Week 1: Foundation

Day 1: Introduction to Somatics

- **Exercise 1**: Diaphragmatic Breathing (3 minutes)
- **Exercise 2**: Body Scan Meditation (5 minutes)
- **Reflection**: Notice sensations in different parts of your body.

Day 2: Gentle Movements

- **Exercise 1**: Somatic Neck Rolls (2 minutes)
- **Exercise 2**: Seated Spinal Twist (3 minutes)
- **Exercise 3**: Mindful Walking (5 minutes)
- **Reflection**: How did the movements affect your posture?

Day 3: Core Awareness

- **Exercise 1**: Pelvic Tilts (2 minutes)
- **Exercise 2**: Abdominal Breathing (3 minutes)
- **Exercise 3**: Bridge Pose (5 minutes)
- **Reflection**: Focus on core engagement during exercises.

Day 4: Grounding Techniques

- **Exercise 1**: Grounding Visualization (3 minutes)
- **Exercise 2**: Standing Tree Pose (3 minutes)

- **Exercise 3**: Legs Up the Wall (4 minutes)
- **Reflection**: Notice sensations of stability and support.

Day 5: Upper Body Relaxation

- **Exercise 1**: Shoulder Rolls (2 minutes)
- **Exercise 2**: Arm Stretches (3 minutes)
- **Exercise 3**: Hand Massage (5 minutes)
- **Reflection**: How did relaxation techniques affect tension?

Day 6: Balance and Coordination

- **Exercise 1**: Single Leg Balance (3 minutes)
- **Exercise 2**: Tai Chi Arm Movements (3 minutes)
- **Exercise 3**: Warrior Pose (4 minutes)
- **Reflection**: Notice improvements in balance.

Day 7: Rest and Restore

- **Exercise 1**: Gentle Stretching (5 minutes)
- **Exercise 2**: Deep Breathing in Child's Pose (5 minutes)
- **Reflection**: Reflect on the week's practices and sensations.

Week 2: Deepening Practice

Day 8: Progressive Muscle Relaxation

- **Exercise 1**: Progressive Muscle Relaxation (5 minutes)
- **Exercise 2**: Full-body Scan (5 minutes)
- **Reflection**: Notice differences in muscle tension.

Day 9: Dynamic Movements

- **Exercise 1**: Dynamic Stretching Routine (5 minutes)

- **Exercise 2**: Flowing Somatic Movements (5 minutes)
- **Reflection**: How did dynamic movements improve flexibility?

Day 10: Joint Mobility

- **Exercise 1**: Joint Rotations (5 minutes)
- **Exercise 2**: Somatic Shoulder Circles (5 minutes)
- **Reflection**: Notice improved range of motion.

Day 11: Mindful Breathing

- **Exercise 1**: Box Breathing (4 minutes)
- **Exercise 2**: Alternate Nostril Breathing (4 minutes)
- **Exercise 3**: Ocean Breath (2 minutes)
- **Reflection**: Focus on breath awareness and relaxation.

Day 12: Core Strength

- **Exercise 1**: Plank Variations (5 minutes)
- **Exercise 2**: Boat Pose (5 minutes)
- **Reflection**: Notice improvements in core stability.

Day 13: Flowing Movements

- **Exercise 1**: Somatic Flow Sequence (7 minutes)
- **Exercise 2**: Dynamic Balance Drills (3 minutes)
- **Reflection**: How did flowing movements improve body awareness?

Day 14: Integrative Rest

- **Exercise 1**: Restorative Yoga Poses (7 minutes)
- **Exercise 2**: Yoga Nidra (3 minutes)
- **Reflection**: Reflect on relaxation techniques.

Week 3: Deep Dive

Day 15: Psoas Release

- **Exercise 1**: Supine Knee-to-Chest Stretch (5 minutes)
- **Exercise 2**: Psoas Self-massage (5 minutes)
- **Reflection**: Notice release in hip and lower back tension.

Day 16: Spinal Alignment

- **Exercise 1**: Cat-Cow Pose (3 minutes)
- **Exercise 2**: Spinal Twists (4 minutes)
- **Exercise 3**: Cobra Pose (3 minutes)
- **Reflection**: Focus on spinal mobility.

Day 17: Stress Relief

- **Exercise 1**: Deep Relaxation Techniques (5 minutes)
- **Exercise 2**: Grounding and Centering (5 minutes)
- **Reflection**: Notice sensations of calmness and relaxation.

Day 18: Mind-Body Awareness

- **Exercise 1**: Body Scan Meditation (5 minutes)
- **Exercise 2**: Mindful Movement Sequence (5 minutes)
- **Reflection**: How does body awareness impact stress levels?

Day 19: Breath and Flow

- **Exercise 1**: Resonance Breathing (5 minutes)
- **Exercise 2**: Somatic Yoga Flow (5 minutes)
- **Reflection**: Notice synchronization of breath and movement.

Day 20: Integration and Alignment

- **Exercise 1**: Feldenkrais Exercises (7 minutes)

- **Exercise 2**: Alignment Drills (3 minutes)

- **Reflection**: How do alignment exercises affect posture?

Day 21: Active Recovery

- **Exercise 1**: Active Stretching Routine (5 minutes)

- **Exercise 2**: Relaxation Techniques (5 minutes)

- **Reflection**: Reflect on recovery benefits.

Week 4: Mastery and Reflection

Day 22: Fluid Movements

- **Exercise 1**: Fluid Somatic Movements (7 minutes)

- **Exercise 2**: Tai Chi Flow (3 minutes)

- **Reflection**: How do fluid movements enhance coordination?

Day 23: Core Integration

- **Exercise 1**: Core Integration Exercises (5 minutes)

- **Exercise 2**: Pilates Core Routine (5 minutes)

- **Reflection**: Notice improved core strength.

Day 24: Mindful Integration

- **Exercise 1**: Mindful Movement Practice (7 minutes)

- **Exercise 2**: Deep Breathing Exercises (3 minutes)

- **Reflection**: How does mindfulness enhance movement?

Day 25: Full-body Awareness

- **Exercise 1**: Full-body Somatic Integration (8 minutes)

- **Exercise 2**: Progressive Relaxation Techniques (2 minutes)

- **Reflection**: Notice overall body awareness.

Day 26: Flow State

- **Exercise 1**: Flowing Somatic Sequences (8 minutes)

- **Exercise 2**: Mindful Walking (2 minutes)

- **Reflection**: Describe sensations of flow and ease.

Day 27: Mastery Practice

- **Exercise 1**: Mastery of Chosen Technique (10 minutes)

- **Reflection**: Reflect on personal growth and achievement.

Day 28: Celebration and Future Planning

- **Exercise 1**: Celebration of Achievements (10 minutes)

- **Reflection**: Set intentions for continued somatic practice.

Adjust exercises based on personal needs and physical abilities. Focus on mindful awareness and gradual progression to maximize benefits from each session.

Week-by-Week Progress Tracker

Scan HERE to download your Tracker !

Video Tutorials

Scan HERE to see the video tutorials of all the exercise !

CONCLUSION
CONTINUING YOUR SOMATIC JOURNEY

Embodying the Lessons Learned

1. Reflection and Integration

- **Reflect Daily**: Take a few moments each day to reflect on insights gained during meditation. Consider how they apply to your thoughts, emotions, and actions.

- **Journaling**: Keep a meditation journal to record your experiences, insights, and any challenges you encountered. Writing can deepen your understanding and commitment to practice.

2. Mindful Awareness Throughout the Day

- **Mindful Activities**: Apply mindfulness to daily activities such as eating, walking, or working. Focus on the present moment, noticing sensations, thoughts, and feelings without judgment.

- **Mindful Breathing**: Use mindful breathing techniques during stressful or challenging situations. Take deep breaths to center yourself and respond consciously rather than reactively.

3. Integrating Mindfulness in Relationships

- **Listening Mindfully**: Practice mindful listening during conversations. Pay attention to the speaker without interrupting or planning your response.

- **Compassionate Communication**: Use mindfulness to cultivate empathy and understanding in your interactions. Respond with kindness and patience.

4. Body-Mind Connection

- **Yoga or Movement Practice**: Incorporate mindful movement practices like yoga or tai chi into your routine. Focus on the sensations in your body and the flow of movement.

- **Body Scan**: Regularly scan your body for areas of tension or discomfort. Practice relaxation techniques to release physical and mental stress.

5. Gratitude and Compassion

- **Gratitude Practice**: Cultivate gratitude by reflecting on what you're thankful for each day. Notice and appreciate the small moments of joy and connection.

- **Self-Compassion**: Be kind to yourself during challenging times. Offer yourself the same compassion you would give to a friend facing difficulty.

6. Continuous Learning and Growth

- **Educate Yourself**: Read books or attend workshops on mindfulness and meditation to deepen your understanding and practice.

- **Community Support**: Engage with a community of practitioners or join meditation groups. Share experiences, insights, and challenges with others on the path.

7. Consistency and Patience

- **Daily Practice**: Maintain a consistent meditation practice, even if it's just a few minutes a day. Consistency builds mindfulness and resilience over time.

- **Patience with Yourself**: Embrace the ups and downs of your journey. Accept that mindfulness is a lifelong practice of growth and discovery.

8. Celebrating Progress

- **Acknowledge Achievements**: Celebrate milestones and progress in your meditation practice. Recognize the positive changes in your life and relationships.

- **Set Intentions**: Regularly revisit your intentions for practicing mindfulness. Adjust them as needed to align with your evolving values and goals.

By embodying the lessons learned from meditation, you cultivate a deeper awareness of yourself and the world around you. This integration fosters resilience, compassion, and a greater sense of well-being in your daily life.

Dear Reader,

Thank you for taking the time to read the first chapter of "Somatic Exercises for Beginners Overcome Stress, Chronic Pain, and Anxiety with 60+ Proven Techniques – a 28-Day Journey to Mind-Body Connection in 10 Minutes a Day | Includes Guided Video Tutorials" Your journey towards better health is important to us, and we hope that the insights provided here have been helpful and inspiring.

Your feedback is invaluable to us. It helps us understand what works well and what can be improved, ensuring that we can provide the best possible content to support you and others on similar paths. By sharing your thoughts, you not only help us improve but also assist other readers in finding the right resources for their needs.

How You Can Share Your Review on Amazon.com:

- Go to the Amazon page where you found my book.
- Navigate to the 'Customer Reviews' section.
- Click on 'Write a customer review' to share your valuable insights.

Instant QR Code Access: Simply scan the QR code below with your smartphone to be directed to the Amazon review section.

www.ingramcontent.com/pod-product-compliance
Lightning Source LLC
Chambersburg PA
CBHW081549250726
48653CB00009B/3346